AROUSAL, ANSWERED

AROUSAL, ANSWERED

An Expert's Guide to Authentic Pleasure and Liberating Sex

KAYNA CASSARD

BLOOMSBURY ACADEMIC
NEW YORK • LONDON • OXFORD • NEW DELHI • SYDNEY

Bloomsbury Publishing Inc, 1359 Broadway, New York, NY 10018, USA
Bloomsbury Publishing Plc, 50 Bedford Square, London, WC1B 3DP, UK
Bloomsbury Publishing Ireland, 29 Earlsfort Terrace, Dublin 2, D02 AY28, Ireland

BLOOMSBURY, BLOOMSBURY ACADEMIC and the Diana logo are
trademarks of Bloomsbury Publishing Plc

First published in the United States of America 2026

Copyright © Kayna Cassard, 2026

Cover design by Jen Hubbert
Front cover image © iStock.com/Carther

All rights reserved. No part of this publication may be: i) reproduced or transmitted in any form, electronic or mechanical, including photocopying, recording or by means of any information storage or retrieval system without prior permission in writing from the publishers; or ii) used or reproduced in any way for the training, development or operation of artificial intelligence (AI) technologies, including generative AI technologies. The rights holders expressly reserve this publication from the text and data mining exception as per Article 4(3) of the Digital Single Market Directive (EU) 2019/790.

Bloomsbury Publishing Inc does not have any control over, or responsibility for, any third-party websites referred to or in this book. All internet addresses given in this book were correct at the time of going to press. The author and publisher regret any inconvenience caused if addresses have changed or sites have ceased to exist, but can accept no responsibility for any such changes.

Library of Congress Cataloging-in-Publication Data

Names: Cassard, Kayna author
Title: Arousal, answered: an expert's guide to authentic pleasure and
liberating sex / Kayna Cassard.
Description: New York: Bloomsbury Academic, 2025. | Includes
bibliographical references and index.
Identifiers: LCCN 2025030501 (print) | LCCN 2025030502 (ebook) |
ISBN 9798881800345 hardback | ISBN 9798881800352 epub |
ISBN 9798765160817
Subjects: LCSH: Sexual excitement | Sex
Classification: LCC HQ31 .C31577 2025 (print) | LCC HQ31 (ebook)
LC record available at https://lccn.loc.gov/2025030501
LC ebook record available at https://lccn.loc.gov/2025030502

ISBN: HB: 979-8-8818-0034-5
ePDF: 979-8-7651-6081-7
eBook: 979-8-8818-0035-2

Typeset by Deanta Global Publishing Services, Chennai, India
Printed and bound in the United States of America

For product safety related questions contact productsafety@bloomsbury.com.

To find out more about our authors and books visit www.bloomsbury.com and
sign up for our newsletters.

CONTENTS

Introduction: How This Book Will Transform Your Sex Life (and Beyond) 1

PART 1 Foundational Necessities 11

1   The Neuroscience for Lifelong Sexual Transformation 15
2   Somatics and Sex 21
3   Sexual Mindfulness 41
4   Cultivating a Pleasure-Based Mindset 55

PART 2 Let's Get Geeky About Your Arousal Potential 75

5   Your Brain: Pathways for Better Arousal and Sex 77
6   Your Body: Sexual Anatomy and Pleasure Science 101
7   Your Energy: Holistic Sexual Wellness 141

PART 3 The Arousal Architecture® 173

8   Your Unique Arousal System 177
9   The Sexual Stimulation Dimension 201
10   The Embodied Experience Dimension 209
11   The Mental Headspace Dimension 217
12   The Energetic Connection Dimension 223
13   The Erotic Exploration Dimension 231
14   Your Arousal Design and Exploration 243

PART 4 Implementation and Application 249

15 How to Use Your New Transformational System in Daily Life 251

16 How to Talk About Sex More Effectively 261

Afterword and Additional Resources 269
Acknowledgments 276
Notes 278
Bibliography 287
Index 296
About the Author 306

Introduction

How This Book Will Transform Your Sex Life (and Beyond)

"So, what do you do?" my ride-share driver asks me. I always take such joy in predicting how this conversation will go. "I'm a sex therapist," I say. Cue the shocked and curious (confused?) look. At this point, they're usually either wondering if I get paid to have sex with clients or if they can get free advice on their current relationship conflict.

I head off misconceptions by explaining further—"I specialize in helping people who have anxiety or pain with sex and the psychological impact it has on them and their relationships." Like most people I tell this to, their eyebrows practically jump off their heads. Sometimes, folks have even shared their surprise that someone could experience emotional or physical pain with sex badly enough that they need to hire a specialist for it. A more shocking number probably realized they're not alone.

Would it surprise *you* if I told you that some researchers estimate that anywhere from 30 percent to 77 percent of people experience some physical or emotional struggle when it comes to sex?[1] The most common among these are issues with sexual desire and arousal. Furthermore, almost 30 percent of women and 41 percent of men in long-term monogamous relationships report feeling sexually dissatisfied in their relationships.[2] As a sex therapist and Educator, I'm both shocked and also not. Most people don't feel comfortable talking about sex, especially if they're having problems with it or wish it were better.

Who do you turn to when problems arise? Most people would think doctors or therapists. However, the likelihood is low that your healthcare providers (or even couples therapists) feel well-versed in the intricacies of troubleshooting sexual challenges from a pleasure-based perspective.

As a result of limited or poor sexual health education, it's no wonder our culture is (not so) secretly obsessed with improving sex. People are aching for self-help information to address the hidden worries that they carry as a daily burden.

When the COVID-19 pandemic struck in 2020, people's lives were upended. Their sex lives weren't immune, either. In a survey conducted by sex researchers, nearly half of the respondents reported a decline in their sex life.[3]

Obviously, people need credible help. That's why it's been my life's work to disrupt the shame-based systems we've all been herded into around sex.

I'm making a solid assumption you want more for your sex life. You know something needs to change. You're tired of believing "that's just how it is." You've probably had a question or two about why your body isn't responding how you think it should (hello, performance anxiety!). This book answers those questions (and more).

I realize that not all folks reading this have had difficulties with sex. If that's you, and you're here to expand your knowledge about sexual arousal and pleasure, I applaud you! We can never stop learning. This book can enhance your sexual experiences and provide you with a more expansive way to understand what you like and how to optimize pleasure with ease and joy.

Plus, you'll learn tools that can improve other areas of your life by reducing stress, anxiety, depression, or relationship conflict.

Regardless of how you feel about sex and arousal, the book you're holding in your hot little hands is your answer to dealing with a lifetime of misinformation, disempowerment, or struggles with sex.

Since 2006, I've been hearing from people about their sexual difficulties, and with my professional training and experience, I've figured out what's needed to overcome the obstacles people often call their "shameful secret." After using the method I'll teach you in this book, clients have learned how to have sexually satisfying lives without pressure, disappointment, or guilt sneaking into their bedrooms uninvited.

Although I've had my own personal experiences of sexual challenges to pull from, you deserve education and guidance based on credible science and research from a professional. As a Licensed Marriage and Family Therapist, Sex Therapist, Certified Trauma Therapist, NeuroSomaticSex Coach™, and Sexual Health Educator, I've been privileged enough to work with thousands of others like you who want to improve their sexual or intimate lives. From their vulnerable stories and our uniquely crafted solutions, I have woven almost two decades of informal clinical research into this book, along with the Arousal Architecture®—the model that will be your key to unlocking more authentic arousal and satisfaction.

As a busy person, I know that when you want to change aspects of your life, part of the challenge is finding time to integrate those changes into your daily routine. With this book, I've taken the essential information you need to know and put it into a "no-fluff" and direct compilation of knowledge and expertise so you can focus on understanding what's happening with your body and sexual response system and initiate changes immediately. You're getting highly specialized insight from a wide range of resources distilled into an easy-to-digest book, so you don't have to spend months (years!) attending therapy with a generalist, sifting through the latest research, or worrying about the accuracy of the information you're getting.

What You're Getting in This Book

My goal with this book is to educate, liberate, and entertain you (at least a little). More specifically, I will help you rewrite sexual narratives and belief systems that are causing you to think your body or sexuality is broken, not normal, or a disappointment.

Part of rewiring our brains for arousal and satisfaction requires rewriting the narrative that "sex should look a certain way" and should happen for only "certain kinds of bodies." Decentering heteronormative, monogamous, "vanilla," and privileged bodies and relationships is not to be taken lightly. These concepts are woven into our society and harm everyone, whether you currently believe that or not.

Throughout this book, you'll see that I include case studies and references to all kinds of bodies, genders, genitalia, and relationship dynamics. I understand if that bumps up against (or even intensely collides with) your belief systems. I hope you will see that I deeply respect people of all types from all walks of life, including folks from conservative, religious, heterosexual, or monogamous belief systems, even as I decenter them.

As such, I've written this content to enable *everyone* to learn something and grow. However, if you find yourself uncomfortable that I refer to examples using pronouns that you don't like or talk about sexual practices that you disagree with, I invite you to use a translator in your fantastic brain and make the switch to something that will help you digest the crucial information.

A note about some gender terms: You will read the words "cisgender" (also "cis man" or "cis woman"). These are people who have been assigned a binary sex that also matches their gender. You might use the term "man" or "woman," but expanding your understanding for more inclusive language around biological sex (e.g., male, female, intersex) and gender is important. I use "men" and "women" when referring to research conducted since that's how the participants identified themselves in the study.

In Part 1, we'll lay the foundation for rewiring your brain's neuropathways to ultimately access or enhance arousal and pleasure. You'll learn to use new perspectives on mindfulness, somatics, and growth mindset concepts and practices as they relate to building a better connection to sexual arousal and pleasure-based sexual practices.

Don't let the emphasis on using these tools for better sex limit your growth—you can use these skills in many more places than the metaphorical bedroom. This book is not only about improving your sexual wellness but also your overall health and well-being.

I've intentionally placed this information first because it helps with the systematic process of getting exposed to sexual content gradually. Learning and practicing these concepts first will start to rewire your brain's neuropathways for feeling more comfortable and confident with creating lasting change and better sex.

Part 2 will be a crash course in pleasure-based sexual health education based on recent peer-reviewed research and sexual science. It's the amount you need without more than you need to know. You'll learn the basics of sexual anatomy, what happens in your brain when sex feels like a threat, and how to rewire neuropathways for arousal and better sex using the science of pleasure.

Since I use a holistic approach to sexual health and wellness, in Part 2, we'll explore the mind-body connection and examine the unique difficulties arising from racism, neurodivergence, and prejudice and the effect those can have on sexual systems and pleasure.

By fully understanding sexual arousal and pleasure anchored in cultural and scientific contexts, you'll see more expansive possibilities for authentic arousal and pleasure instead of dwelling in shame spirals that there's something inherently wrong with you or your sexual self.

With your brain and body ready for new pathways, in Part 3, I'll introduce you to a powerful model and system I developed for people just like you called the Arousal Architecture®. You'll also learn expansive and practical techniques that have been helping my clients for years.

Although I initially created the Arousal Architecture® for people who have had challenges with sex and arousal, it can also help anyone who wants to uncover new and unique ways to become aroused. If you're familiar with the concepts of Love Languages®, it's similar, but for your arousal system. You'll learn your *arousal language.*

The Arousal Architecture® is your new and empowering tool to disrupt oppressive systems that have historically suppressed sexual pleasure and arousal. It's the model you need, regardless of how much sex you have, want to have, or who you're having it with.

In Part 4, you'll have the opportunity to explore and utilize resources immediately to help you integrate what you learn from this book. We'll identify regular practices you can incorporate into your life more quickly than you think. You'll find exercises and interventions for everyone and in a wide variety of situations—flying solo, dating, or in a committed partnership with one or more people. Additionally, I've created some practical resources, such as communication formulas and strategies for talking to healthcare providers about sexual health needs, to help you continue to expand your new sexual narrative with confidence.

How to Get the Most from This Book

Contrary to what you might expect, this book doesn't begin with topics that are explicitly about "the juicy stuff." I do this for a few reasons. First, if sex feels weighted with physically or emotionally painful experiences, diving headfirst into talking about pleasure or explicitly sexual content can make it challenging to incorporate the lessons on a deeper level. I witnessed the transformative power of structuring my online courses, intensives, psychotherapy, and coaching programs using the NeuroSomaticSex Method™ for Sex Therapy and Coaching, so I employed a similar approach in this book.

Second, it's essential to prepare your nervous system (your mind and body) by understanding what to do when information (like pleasure-based sexual education) is overwhelming, scary, or uncomfortable. You may encounter topics in this book that make you want to set it down, promising to read it later. Months later, you've forgotten about it and are back to old patterns of avoiding arousal problems and wondering why your sex life hasn't changed.

When sex is painful (physically or emotionally), we collude with our brains to avoid it. It's natural. That's why I've structured the book the way I have. I'm your guide in disrupting those avoidance patterns.

Case Studies

Throughout the book, I've included *Case Studies* to provide real-life examples from my clients (identifying information has been changed for privacy), my own experiences, and others who have generously shared their experiences with me to help others like you learn and grow.

Going Deeper Exercises

Within the chapters, you'll find suggested exercises for experiential practices that will create an immersive experience as you read.

If you'd like to try some of the exercises but not others, no problem. If you don't want to do any of them, that's also okay! While everything in here is designed to give you what I know is the most helpful, you are the expert in you. I trust that you will use what you need. If you're not going to engage in the exercise, at least read through it, because it can still create powerful change simply by exposing you to the content.

Quick Win! Exercises

Some folks wish they had the time and energy to do all the exercises but just can't fit them in, no matter how hard they try. I've included *Quick Wins!* throughout the book for this exact reason.

I call them *Quick Wins!* because simply doing them is a win. It's not about the goal or outcome; it's about engaging in something that attempts to create shifts, even if that's one degree or percentage of change. Something is better than nothing if you hope to change the current state of things.

Pleasure Gems

At the end of relevant chapters, you'll find a section titled "Pleasure Gems" to highlight the most important information discussed.

By revisiting the *Pleasure Gems* and exercises regularly, you can enhance your knowledge and growth. Each time you finish a chapter, I invite you to re-read the *Pleasure Gems* of the chapters you've already read. This will help refresh your memory on the content and key points covered. It will also keep the topics in mind, which will continue to rewire your pathways for reinforcing more impactful and sustained change.

Perfectionism Is the Kryptonite for Growth

Don't let perfectionism get in the way of moving forward. Speaking from experience, I know how easy it is to get overwhelmed and stalled by exercises I don't have time for. That's why I wanted to make my book different.

It will be better to move forward in learning and doing what you can than to hold yourself back from trying to do everything perfectly in a particular order. Be kind and realistic with yourself. Take what resonates and leave the rest. If you're getting stuck on something more often than moving forward, reach out so I can help you figure out the culprit keeping you stuck and find sustainable solutions for accountability and creating change.

Emotional Overwhelm and Trauma Activation

When it comes to sex, knowing that a traumatic experience or a history of trauma is a part of your story can be overwhelming, scary, or challenging to want to engage in anything related to sex. You have every right to decide to pause on your sexual wellness journey and this book. It will be here for you when you're ready.

In other cases, you might not know of any past trauma, but you still feel emotionally activated as you read. Some folks can be triggered or dissociate without realizing it. This might be experienced as floaty sensations, feeling numb or disconnected from your body, or noticing tension, anxiety, or fear.

Chapters 2 and 3 incorporate trauma-informed practices that can help you navigate moments when you feel dysregulated but still want to continue reading. Refer to those as frequently as you need. It's the main reason why they're at the beginning of the book, so you learn them immediately.

The goal is to arrive back in your body in a way that doesn't feel out of control, however you define that. If you're not able to achieve regulation well enough to continue, it's essential to have a professional qualified to work with trauma. There are resources at the back of this book that can help you find assistance.

I also offer a free resource on my website, called the "Mindfulness First Aid Kit," which you can download and use as you read through the book. Find it at www.cassardcenter.com/freebies.

Get Ready to Have Your Questions about *Arousal, Answered*

I know you're here because you desire sexual satisfaction and new tools that make arousal and sex more manageable and more joyful. You've been looking for answers as to why you've felt anxious, guilty, disappointed, or ashamed of how arousal or sex shows up in your life. Regardless of your experience, I deeply empathize with you. I've lived with struggles myself, having suffered from painful sex for over a decade. It damaged my sexual self-esteem, shut down my arousal system, and challenged my self-confidence in such intense ways that I often doubted I would ever feel sexually whole and happy.

If you resonate with even a smidge of that, this book will provide you with tools to bounce back when things get tough, rather than spiraling into catastrophic thinking and shutting down. *Arousal, Answered* is the culmination of the central resources I found invaluable to claiming potent sexual resiliency and intimate satisfaction. It's also what my clients use to overcome their sexual challenges with confidence.

And now it's your turn.

By the end of this book, I hope that you'll walk away with a new perspective on your sexuality and sexual functioning, armed with powerful techniques, exercises, and a more effective way to talk about (and have) sex.

Welcome to *Arousal, Answered*—your exciting and expertly led guide to solutions for challenging questions about authentic arousal and liberating sex.

PART 1

FOUNDATIONAL NECESSITIES

Before diving into sexual health and pleasure, we'll start with some foundational concepts related to mindfulness, somatics, and mindset.

You might be thinking, "This is a sexual health book, so why are we not talking about sex and pleasure right away?" Trust me, there's a reason.

Learning this information and practicing techniques in low-pressure situations (such as non-sexual activities) prepares you for moments that feel more important or have more pressure (like sex). This way, when you're ready to address your sexual life directly, you'll have the skills and confidence to handle it.

Embarking on the journey of confronting and changing long-held sexual challenges or negative beliefs is not an easy task. You might be tempted to hide this book away and forget about it.

However, that discomfort you feel is a sign that you're on the path to personal growth. Our brains are wired to prefer the status quo, even if it means continuing with sexual dissatisfaction. This resistance is your brain's way of alerting you to an important area for change. Just focus on the next step rather than the entire journey.

Your next step in the following chapters is learning how neuroscience-rooted concepts in somatics (body-based practices), mindfulness, and growth mindsets will help you incorporate popular and effective techniques into your bedroom escapades. And here's a bonus: These skills also apply beyond sexual wellness, helping reduce stress, increase happiness, and improve areas like financial stability and career satisfaction.[1]

Even if you don't have sexual challenges, the tools in the following chapters are phenomenal for optimizing sex and improving quality of life.

My Journey and Why It Matters

Before we go any further, I'd like to tell you a little about where the concept of this book started because that journey provides context for why the following chapters differ from what you'll likely find in other sexual self-help books.

Since 2006, I've been immersed in the sexual health field, understanding the wide range of struggles people face. I began as a Sexual Health Educator, teaching others to release shame-based education and embrace pleasure-based practices. But I wanted to go deeper and help people heal on a foundational level.

During this time, I faced my own sexual challenges: hormone-mediated vulvodynia and vaginismus. These conditions, caused by factors like birth control, sex-negative messages, and trauma, led to fear of sex, low libido, and damaged sexual self-esteem. Despite my education, I realized pleasure-based sex education alone wasn't enough for lasting healing. Sexual challenges lasting longer than six months or causing clinical distress require more than simply learning the mechanics of how to have more pleasurable sex.

Through my work as a Licensed Marriage and Family Therapist, Sex Therapist, Painful Sex Specialist, and Certified Trauma Therapist, I've helped thousands find lasting change. However, traditional psychotherapy with specialized sex therapists is often slow and costly. Determined to find a better way, I delved into business courses, coaching programs, and mentorships, eventually becoming the CEO of my company, Sex, Answered.

The concepts I learned to grow my business surprisingly also applied to improving sex and intimacy, leading to profound insights and changes around the traditional sex therapy or education model. This revelation helped me create more effective and accessible sexual wellness and treatment programs.

I found the final missing pieces in creating change that didn't burn clients out from traditional psychotherapy, reducing treatment time and making it more financially accessible to many more people.

Combined with all my professional, educational, and business experiences, I created sexual wellness and treatment programs in my clinical practice that were structured differently than anything else I saw being offered.

I've crafted the information in this book similarly to these program models. Consider this book an overview of the more extensive programs I help private clients through. I hope that *Arousal, Answered* creates one more level of accessible aid for people to gain specialized education and support.

Ready for your next step? Let's explore how neuroscience, mindfulness, somatics, and a growth mindset can transform your overall wellness and sexual life.

1

The Neuroscience for Lifelong Sexual Transformation

Neuroscience may not sound sexy—but it's the secret to unlocking wild, authentic pleasure over a lifetime. But don't worry, if the idea of reading about science makes your eyes immediately glaze over, I'll only cover what you absolutely need to know to make sex more enjoyable. Neuroscience focuses on the structure of the brain and nervous system and how they function, informed by a wide range of scientific studies, perspectives, and research, including neurochemistry, experimental psychology, anatomy, and developmental biology.

Speaking simply, the goal of this book is to get you from one place (less satisfying sex) to a different place (more satisfying sex). This doesn't just occur in some magical way. You have a lot more control over it than you might realize. Science can explain a lot about why we act, feel, and think in certain ways, which can reduce the shame that's often tied to believing there's something inherently wrong with us when sex doesn't work the way we expect it to.

Neuroscience answers a lot of questions about sex for people, especially the question, "What's wrong with me?" When my clients learn that repeated or intense experiences can influence the way that their body responds in sexual situations, they understand that it's a result of a changeable neuroscientific process, instead of feeling shame because they think they're broken or weird. They also learn they can have more control over the process and begin to craft the kind of sex life they prefer to have.

Learning about neuroscience and how it impacts sex and arousal helps demystify the process and makes it more tangible. Most people typically think that a "sex drive" is something you have, or you don't. Many people also think that the act of being physiologically aroused (indicated by lubrication, erection, etc.) is something that should happen naturally or when all the stars align in the right way. When folks learn that they can have a lot more influence on their arousal, interests, and experiences, it inspires more confidence and excitement. Sex and sexual arousal aren't some random, undefined experiences that happen naturally to people (or not). You can learn how to actively engage in creating empowering sexual experiences with more ease. Neuroscience helps you find the way through and lays out the path for change. It's the most essential perspective for satisfying sexual wellness, in my opinion.

Neuroscience for Learning and Unlearning Behaviors and Outdated Beliefs

Now let's examine how we learn from a neurobiological perspective. This will help you understand how mindfulness, somatic practices, and a growth mindset can fit into your transformative process. The following information is a quick overview of a very complex process that will help you without getting too deep into the weeds.

Almost everything we know, particularly as it relates to sex, has been learned over time. *Factual knowledge* about life (such as how to tie your shoe or the practical process of having sex) and our *beliefs* are not innate. You are not born with *most* factual knowledge, and you do not have most of the belief systems about the world or yourself built into your little mind and body when you're born. You learn these things as you grow and interact with the world.

For this discussion, *belief systems* are sets of ideas strung together to form opinions about intimacy, relationships, and sex that seem like factual truth or "just the way it is." Sometimes, what you learn and begin to believe is based on outdated information or an agenda that conflicts with what feels good or right to you, especially as an adult. We'll talk in depth about this in Part 2 to make it a lot more tangible and specifically related to sex. For now, the most important thing to know is that when you have lived a few decades learning explicitly or implicitly about sex, you're likely going to come up against belief systems that were helpful at one point (like the need to abstain from sex before marriage, or that "boys" like "girls," etc.) but are not helping now because your life circumstances, cognitive beliefs, or sexuality have shifted, and they're no longer in alignment. When that happens, internal conflict arises consciously or subconsciously. Subsequently, sexual issues and challenges can occur, creating barriers to the kind of sex and intimacy you want to have but can't figure out why it's not easier.

Creating awareness about your belief systems and behavioral reactions is the first step in the Sexual Wellness Neuroscience Formula:

Self-Awareness + Unlearning + Rewiring = Authentic Sexual Wellness

We'll get into how to deepen sexual self-awareness later, so for now we'll stay focused on the crucial understanding that sexual challenges and barriers are *learned responses*. By believing that a sexual issue is a learned response, you can develop more authentic sexual wellness through the process of "unlearning" and "rewiring" behavioral responses and belief systems around sex, arousal, and pleasure.

It is especially important to comprehend the process of learned responses when dealing with something that has been emotionally or physically painful, like a profoundly disappointing attempt at having pain-free sex or accidentally touching a hot stove that you thought was off.

Let's say that when you engage in some behavior (e.g., touching a stove, having sex, etc.), undesirable consequences happen every time (or almost every time). As a result, your brain and body will form a belief system about that behavior. Then, when you're presented with an opportunity to touch a stove or have sex, your nervous system will send "alert" signals to be cautious or even afraid because you've always (or almost always) experienced something unpleasant paired with that event.

This unpleasant process typically results in muscle tension, changes in our brain function to focus on safety, and the release of chemicals in our bodies that gear us up to fight, flee, freeze, or fawn. This often shuts down sexual arousal, creating a limited desire for sex or even difficulty reaching orgasm.

You can conceptualize this in a simple formula:

Event + Unpleasant Consequence = Threat = Aversion/Avoidance

Hopefully, you're starting to see that if you've had challenges with sex in the past, it's not likely about who you are as a sexual person or partner. Instead, exposure to sex-negative information and possibly painful or harmful experiences has created learned responses that reinforce that sex and arousal are ultimately unpleasant.

Now, let's say you haven't had belief systems, repeated unpleasant experiences, or trauma that get in your way of sex (or at least not that you're aware of at this point). You might be reading this book because you think sex and arousal have lost their luster. Or you're simply tired from daily chores, working, and caring for a home or family, and sex feels less satisfying than it once did. There is still a process of learning and unlearning that happens with those experiences, too. As much as you hate to admit it, moments for intimacy, sex, or connection can feel like one more expectation to deal with, and you just don't have it in you. That's completely normal, and it doesn't mean anything's wrong with you, your partner, or your relationship. This is also a learned response. This book will assist you in finding low-energy ways to unlearn that process so you can stop feeling like sex is just another chore or obligation on your to-do list.

Similarly, people in long-term, committed, monogamous relationships will often express feeling like they've lost the spark they had at the beginning of their relationship. Usually, this happens after anywhere from the first six months to about a year and a half. I'm sure you've heard of the "honeymoon phase," when it can feel much easier to be organically aroused by or feel desire for your partner. We'll dive more into this phenomenon in Part 2, but right now, I hope you can find comfort in the fact that barriers to spontaneous arousal and sex can be normal and, in many cases, are learned responses that can be unlearned!

Even when a thought, belief, or feeling seems automatic or unchangeable, it's not entirely the case if you don't want it to be. Neuroscience (and sometimes somatic sex therapy) can be a beneficial tool when people have difficulty with sex and don't want it to be the way it is but don't know how to change it.

One of the most essential concepts in this book is "neuroplasticity." Neuroplasticity is your brain's ability to learn responses and change them to a more desirable process. It helps us understand that we can influence how our brain is structured and processes information received from the world around us.[1] This means that doors are now opening for you with new opportunities around thinking, acting, and feeling simply by learning how to make your brain and body work *for* you rather than *against* you.

Pleasure Gems

- Belief systems are typically learned responses, meaning you can use your brain's neuroplastic capabilities to alter belief systems into something that aligns with what makes you feel good and with your present-day values.

- The Sexual Wellness Neuroscience Formula gives us a framework for creating change. It includes a process of self-awareness along with unlearning outdated belief systems and rewiring new experiences, which will facilitate authentic sexual and overall wellness.

- By understanding that learned responses contribute to many sexual challenges and that neuroscience can be used to rewrite neuropathways, you're starting to bust the guilt-shame spiral.

- You're not broken; you learned about sex in a broken system, and this book can help you rewrite your sexual narrative.

2

Somatics and Sex

My favorite tool for rewiring brain pathways and learning new concepts or behaviors is the practice of somatics. I often get confused looks from other professionals and clients alike when I mention "somatics" as it relates to sex therapy and coaching. So, in case you're also unsure about what I mean, let's get clear on some definitions first:

- *Somatics*, for the purposes of this book, is the practice of creating awareness of one's body and the present-moment, especially by focusing on bodily sensations or movement to improve mental health.
- *Somatic therapies* are healing modalities and practices that help people release emotions and, in some cases, reprocess trauma using various mind-body techniques.
- The *mind-body connection* process is a two-way "conversation" between your mind and body, where the mind influences the body and the body influences the mind.

The power of using the body to heal is not a new concept—it's been a healing practice for thousands of years in Eastern, Asian, Latin, African, and Indigenous cultures. You might be familiar with some of these practices, such as yoga, styles of dance, Reiki, meditation, drumming, tai chi, and qi gong. Westerners and colonizers brought various somatic practices to the West

(Europe and North America), altering and appropriating them into modern-day Western modalities. Although going into the origins of these practices is beyond the scope of this book, it's important to honor, acknowledge, and provide reparation in welcomed and meaningful ways around the benefits that many of us white therapists, coaches, and other Western healers have gained from the appropriation of these practices.

The term "somatics" was coined in the 1970s in the West, with the popularity of Somatic Experiencing, which was developed in the same decade.[1] Although incorporating somatic practices into sex therapy has been increasing in popularity in the last few years, I've been using it as a core component in my practice since 2015 for a good reason—it works on a level that typical talk therapy doesn't quite reach.

"Talk therapy" is the practice of psychotherapy that mainly relies on a client and therapist talking about emotions, mental health struggles, or past experiences, along with identifying insights, revelations, or solutions that hopefully help resolve the client's challenges.

Compare this to "somatic therapy," which engages the body in psychotherapy sessions alongside talk therapy, inviting the client to notice sensations occurring in the body or moving the body in ways to help release stuck emotions or energy.

Since there wasn't a lot of research on somatic psychotherapy when I was a brand-spankin' new therapist in 2011, it wasn't a modality commonly taught in many Clinical Psychology programs like mine. Ironically, I didn't get my first exposure to somatic healing from anything directly related to my studies in psychology. Instead, I realized there was power in "bringing the body" into the therapeutic conversation when I explored a hobby called acroyoga.

This practice blends yoga, partner acrobatics, and Thai massage together as a playful and fun form of exercise. My hobby (read: obsession) developed into a proficient practice. Eventually, I began moonlighting as an international acroyoga instructor, leading intimacy retreats and incorporating this passion with my professional expertise.

I started to see the power of using one's body, trust, and connection to another to heal experiences that were hard to treat using talk therapy alone. So many of my fellow "acroyogis" shared their profound healing experiences beyond the practice as a recreational sport.

As a teacher and practitioner of acroyoga, I kept hearing stories from others talking about the transformative experiences from acroyoga (and even yoga). I knew I also needed to bring these concepts to my psychotherapy clients. I dove into reading well-known body-based trauma healing books like *Waking the Tiger*, *The Body Keeps the Score*, *My Grandmother's Hands*, and *Trauma and the Body*, and focused my clinical attention on becoming a Certified Trauma Therapist from the Trauma Resource Institute—a center whose trauma treatment education and trainings are based in neuroscience and somatic experiences.[2]

The impact of bringing this work into the practice of sex therapy blew my mind as I saw my clients overcome their sexual challenges much quicker than when we used the gold standard cognitive behavioral therapy (CBT) and traditional talk therapy methods. Even though a ton of research supports CBT as an effective sex therapy, my clients were having many more breakthroughs with the somatic practices and trauma reprocessing methods I was trained in.

I was sold: Somatics would be part of my work moving forward, including incorporating it into standard sex therapy CBT practices. Not only did I see a profound change in my psychotherapeutic practice, but I also experienced the transformation myself in my own healing journey as I learned to cultivate the language of my body and use it to heal sexual pain and improve how I experienced authentic pleasure.

And now, it's your turn to learn how somatic practices can help you create easier access to your arousal and improved sexual experiences using the foundational practices you'll find in this chapter. Then, you'll build on them for enhanced sexual wellness as you read this book.

Why Somatics Improve Sex

When I was first exposed to somatic practices and experienced profound healing, I thought it was pure magic. The scientist in me needed to know why they worked, and surprise, surprise, the answers were rooted in neuroscience.

As we explored, seemingly automatic behaviors and beliefs evolve through learned responses. If you want to change how you think, feel, or respond to situations, especially as it relates to sex or situations that hijack your nervous system, simply telling yourself to change is not as effective as helping your body learn how to believe in the transformation you wish to achieve.

When clients express frustration around *wanting* to want sex, or when they're attracted to their partners but their bodies don't cooperate, that's when weaving somatics into our work is essential to helping them achieve their goals for more satisfying sex.

Not only do somatic practices assist in rewiring the brain and belief systems, but they can also regulate the nervous system and reduce anxiety. As a result, this improves your mind-body connection so you can learn new concepts and behaviors to create healthier brain pathways. Being more regulated or calm makes learning quicker and easier than being in an anxious or disconnected state.

By doing this, you're making friends with your body, so it works *for* you rather than *against* you, especially when figuring out how you want to experience better sex, arousal, and pleasure.

Introductory Somatic Healing Practices to Try

There is a wide variety of systems and models based in somatics that healers and therapists use to help their clients. At Sex, Answered we use EMDR (Eye Movement Desensitization and Reprocessing) Sex Therapy and the

NeuroSomaticSex Method™ for Therapy and Coaching which, as you might guess, combines neuroscience and somatic practices, along with a few other components that you'll find woven throughout this book. Many other powerful somatic therapies exist, such as Somatic Experiencing, Sensorimotor Psychotherapy, and Somatic Attachment.[3] There are also bodywork practices based on somatics, such as Myofascial Release, the Alexander Technique, and Rolfing.[4]

Many somatic modalities are rooted in neuroscience and the understanding that our bodies hold tension around unpleasant experiences. Healing comes from identifying where energy (in the form of a body response or reaction) is located or stuck, then helping the body release or move that energy. This is particularly impactful for recurring unpleasant or harmful experiences (like oppressive belief systems or trauma) or ones that feel shameful, such as disappointing or painful sex.

The following information and somatic practices skim the surface. Still, I believe they are usually enough for most people to start the process of improving sexual arousal and pleasure. If you find that it's not enough to reach your sexual well-being goals, it could be helpful to seek out a specialized professional to support you with deeper somatic techniques.

I start somatic healing with my clients by teaching them about their bodies' language (a.k.a. sensations). Knowing what to look for and how to describe what you're experiencing can be tricky when you're starting to learn and utilize your body's language, despite seeming obvious.

Let's take a very surface-level look at a common example to understand the process involving emotions and sensations.

Imagine you're on a walk in the forest, and suddenly, you see a mountain lion. The first emotion you probably feel is fear, and then your brain has determined you're faced with a threat. Your brain sends signals to your body to prepare it to brace for an attack, fight, or run away to keep you safe (I'm referring to the flight/fight response). In trauma work, there are other reactions that our bodies have when confronted with fear (like fawning or freezing), but since this book is trauma-informed and not trauma reprocessing, we'll stick to the basics for now.

So, when your body faces a threat, it prepares to keep you safe by acting on messages from your brain to turn off certain bodily functions that are unnecessary for survival (such as digestion or sexual arousal). Simultaneously, the brain activates the parts of your body like major muscle groups that are necessary to brace, run, or fight. This process of nervous system activation results in different sensations occurring throughout your body as parts of it turn on or off, such as increased muscle tension or heart rate.

When your nervous system determines the threat is over, in the best-case scenario, it becomes more regulated, and a reverse process occurs. As a result, different sensations arise as body systems (like digestion) are turned on and muscle tension or activation is turned off. Typical sensations during this process are relaxed muscles, deeper breaths, or a gurgling stomach.

Not all "threats" are mountain lions. When it comes to sex, threats could be physical pain like vulvodynia, endometriosis, or vaginismus. Threats can be in the form of emotional pain, such as guilt, pressure, shame, or disappointment when dealing with low arousal, erectile variabilities, or orgasm difficulties. If you experience those emotions with sex, your brain can interpret "sex" as a "threat," causing nervous system activation and subsequent body sensations that feel like shutting down or avoidance.

We'll discuss this in more depth in Part 2, but the main point is that our bodies often experience sensations simultaneously when we have thoughts, emotions, or face a threat. The sensations might be subtle or blatantly obvious, but they're almost always there. Most people don't realize this is happening just under the surface of their awareness. Before doing somatic work, my clients often express feeling "cut off from their bodies" or like they're "floating heads." You learn your body's language by developing an awareness of the sensations that occur within you as you move through your day. By noticing and distinguishing between sensations of anxiety versus regulation versus joy, for example, you can have more control over how you experience different scenarios. This is one way to "be embodied." The more embodied you are, the easier it becomes to influence your sexual arousal system and overcome sexual anxieties or pain instead of being hijacked by them.

Exploring Sensations: Your Body's Language

You're now going to build self-awareness and embodiment by exploring sensations, which contribute to the Sexual Wellness Neuroscience Formula.

First, instead of thinking about what you're experiencing as negative versus positive, which might imply a judgment about it (thereby creating unnecessary tension), you can adapt your language to using "pleasant," "neutral," or "unpleasant." This is especially helpful when exploring sensations because they're not inherently bad; they're informative about what's happening in your body physiologically.

In a few pages, you'll find a Sensations List to help you with the basics. Not everyone is the same, so this is just a starting point for understanding how your body *might* respond in various situations. Take what works for you, add to it, and leave what doesn't resonate!

It's important to note that "neutral" is different from "numb." *Neutral* is an experience of a part of your body (or something happening with your body) that isn't unpleasant and might not be precisely pleasant either (although people often describe neutral as enjoyable, too).

For example, if you have a pinky (not everyone does), you might sense that it's attached to your body. You notice sensations that are not unpleasant, nor are they pleasant, but it's simply existing and present in your awareness.

Sometimes, neutral can be the absence of an unpleasant sensation, such as the absence of tension when you might typically feel tension in your chest.

Alternatively, *numb* is a lack of sensation or connection to your body or part of your body. It can also be felt as cold, disconnected, or floaty.

Regularly experiencing numbness or overwhelmingly unpleasant sensations could indicate a need for a specialized professional to provide somatically based trauma response regulation or trauma reprocessing, even if you don't have any identifiable traumas that you're aware of.

Sensations are descriptive experiences of what's happening in the body. They're not "feelings" or "emotions," although most of my clients usually confuse the two when they first start these practices. As an example, you might feel the emotion of anxiety, but think about how you *know* it's anxiety in your body. What sensations accompany anxiety?

Sensations can also differ from person to person. For instance, in a support group I lead for overcoming painful sex and sexual avoidance, one of the group members explained she feels anxiety as tightness in her chest. On the other hand, another one shared that she mainly feels nausea in her stomach and unpleasant energy stuck in her arms. There's no right or wrong, only what is.

Now that you know about possible sensations you may experience, you can try the following exercises to build self-awareness and engage in nervous system regulation techniques to help you become more embodied. This will help with rewiring your brain pathways when confronted with unpleasant responses to addressing outdated belief systems and overcoming sexual barriers. The more you can get your nervous system to a regulated state (meaning when you generally feel neutral or at least not hijacked by unpleasant sensations), the easier it will be to learn the information in this book and effectively use the powerful processes for changing your relationship to sexual arousal and pleasure.

Although noticing sensations seems simple, listening to your body's language can be quite difficult. It's similar to learning any other language—you must practice and be kind to yourself because this might be uncharted territory. If you're overwhelmed by trying to notice all the possible sensations, start by focusing on noticing your muscles, heart rate, or breathing. Narrowing it down to those three will help you become accustomed to your body and its response to thoughts or situations.

Start with these somatic practices in everyday experiences. Then, in Part 2, you'll learn how to apply them to sexual contexts.

SENSATIONS LIST

Sensations typically felt with *unpleasant emotions or situations*:

- Muscle or overall body tension
- Constricted or shallow breathing
- Fast heart rate
- Nausea
- Heaviness
- Skin crawling
- Shaky
- Dizzy
- Itching
- Lightheaded
- Hollow
- Dull

Sensations typically associated with *neutral or pleasant emotions or experiences*:

- Calm
- Lightness
- Tingling
- Expansion or openness
- Deeper or easier breaths
- Relaxed muscles
- Energized
- Movement
- Grounded
- Regular or slowed heart rate

Somatic Practice: Sensation Snapshot

This process will help you develop self-awareness and is a significant initial step toward building more emotional and sexual resiliency. In this exercise, you "take a snapshot" of the sensations occurring in your body at this moment. You can do this in various ways.

One easy and straightforward way is to ask yourself what sensations grab your attention in any given moment. This technique is handy when you feel a strong emotion, like anxiety or guilt, and especially pleasure or joy. You can also use it in the reverse: when you notice sensations that occur, they can help you identify the feelings you usually associate with them. To do this, when you have a feeling or experience a situation that elicits a response in your body, ask yourself, "What sensations are strongest right now?" Or "What do I notice happening in my body right now?"

Another option is to perform a body scan, starting at the top of your head, "tracking" or noticing sensations as you move through your body to your toes.[5]

As you read the following, I invite you to engage in this exercise with me. However, if paying attention to your body's sensations is not something you want to do, that's not a problem—you do you! Either read through it to understand how the process might sound in your head or skip to the next exercise.

If you do this exercise now or in the future, remember that there's no right or wrong way to do it. Release any expectation that it should look a certain way. You might not notice anything close to the suggestions or descriptions I provide; they are just examples to inspire ideas around what you might experience. Remember, be kind to yourself too. If you become distracted and feel too much "in your head," simply redirect your focus back to the present moment and try to get embodied again.

Here we go.

Starting at the top of your head, notice whether you're holding tension in your jaw, in other places, or not at all. Do you notice other sensations in or on your face? Maybe your nose is a little cold, or you feel the warm pressure of your tongue on the roof of your mouth.

As you move to your neck and shoulders, what do you notice? Is there a lump in your throat, does it feel constricted, or does it feel open? Are your shoulders dropping away from your ears or are they tight toward the sky?

Continue down into your chest and arms. Notice if there's movement of energy or stagnation. Do you feel your fingers tingly, wishing to be shaken out? Or maybe this part of your body feels primarily neutral. Perhaps you notice a heaviness somewhere in the core of your body.

As you shift toward your pelvic area, what sensations attract your attention? Does it feel numb or disconnected here (as it does with many people with sexual challenges)? Or maybe you feel connected to your sexual wellness, and you feel warmth or pleasant tingles here.

Continue to notice the sensations that grab your attention as you move your focus to your hips, legs, and knees. Do you feel tension or pain here? Maybe they're sore from a workout. Or perhaps you notice strength and powerful energy.

As you direct your attention to your feet and toes, notice the sensations here, such as grounded, tingles, coolness, or heat.

If you're following along with your body while reading, I invite you to notice your overall feelings and sensations. Do you feel better, worse, different, or about the same as when you started? This isn't a pop quiz, and I don't have an expectation of what you "should" feel; this is just an invitation to notice how things might have changed after the exercise.

Now, let's take a breath and prepare to shift back to the cognitive process of continuing to read and learn.

Somatic Practice: Redirect to Neutral or Pleasant

The previous exercise aimed to help you notice *any* sensations occurring in your body. With the Redirecting to Neutral or Pleasant exercise, the goal is pretty simple: refocus your attention from unpleasant sensations to neutral or pleasant ones. That's it.

As with most of what we've discussed, the instructions might be simple, but practicing the exercise might be much more difficult.

This exercise is designed to help you with two things: nervous system regulation and building (or reinforcing) brain pathways that align with how you want to feel, think, or experience situations, particularly sexually pleasurable ones.

I teach this exercise after the Sensation Snapshot because if you notice unpleasant sensations or emotions in your body while doing that exercise, you can switch to the Redirecting to Neutral or Pleasant exercise. You can also use it in any other unpleasant experience or situation that occurs. In that case, instead of first checking in with your body to see what's happening, you can focus immediately on neutral or pleasant sensations.

Sometimes, locating neutral or pleasant sensations can be difficult when you're in a bad mood, feeling anxious, or having any other unpleasant experience. Having a tried-and-tested "anchor" can be really helpful here. A "neutral anchor" is a place in your body that tends to be reliably neutral. Common neutral body parts include the tip of the nose, earlobe, or pinky fingernail. Many of my clients choose their feet because they are usually the farthest from unpleasant sensations or emotions experienced in their bodies. Regularly using the Sensation Snapshot to create more embodied self-awareness can help you locate places that are typically neutral in your body.

Somatic Practice: Noticing Pleasant

If you feel like you're mastering your focus on neutral, or you want to build more joy and "non-sexual" pleasure, practice my favorite tool, Noticing Pleasant, where you seek pleasant sensations as often as possible. Weaving an emphasis on pleasure into your daily life and as regularly as possible makes being mindful and present much more effortless. Plus, when we constantly strive to notice pleasant sensations, we're actively working to regulate our nervous systems, increasing our well-being overall. Health and wellness pave the way for delicious sexual arousal.

Noticing pleasant sensations differs significantly from toxic positivity, such as the "good vibes only" concept. Your goal in seeking pleasure (especially "non-sexual" pleasure) is not about ignoring or shoving down unpleasant sensations, emotions, or thoughts. Instead, aim to notice moments of pleasure or joy whenever you can, even if you're also having unpleasant experiences.

For instance, you might have just hung up from a bothersome phone call with a friend while you're on a walk during spring when the trees and plants are sprouting new growth. Instead of toxic positivity that tells us to "just get over the upsetting conversation or forget it happened and move on," you can recognize that you feel upset about the conversation and honor the emotions and thoughts arising. Simultaneously, you're also aware of how it feels in your body when you look at the beauty of the little leaf sprouts and the new flower buds starting to pop out around you. Even though you're bothered by the call with your friend, you're *also* noticing places in your body where you can sense pleasant responses by focusing on the present moment around you.

With time, as you are able to redirect to pleasant more than neutral, your resiliency for tolerating emotional discomfort or managing pain will be much more powerful. It will help you gently push up against the edge of resistance in a regulated and safe way, helping you get out of your comfort zone and try new things or create alternative possibilities and opportunities.

Plus, when it comes to increasing sexual arousal and pleasure, when you start to create brain pathways that know how to seek and experience pleasurable sensations, it will be much easier for you to activate sexual arousal and sexual satisfaction. The structure of this book is intentionally designed to start with practicing these skills in lower-pressure situations first. That way, you already feel familiar with using the skill in situations where outcomes feel a lot more important to you, like having solo or partnered sex.

By practicing in non-sexual situations, you're setting yourself up for success in more anxiety-provoking sexual situations in the future. Your body learns the metaphorical muscle memory of these practiced somatic techniques, leaving you with more resources to focus on being present and enjoying sexual play when the time comes.

Be kind to yourself through these practices. Use curiosity around your experiences and avoid judging or criticizing what happens. We'll talk more in depth about how to do that soon.

When to Use Somatic Practices

As mentioned, you learn best when in a regulated and open headspace. The previous practices and others mentioned in this part of the book will help you cultivate nervous system regulation, thereby creating a more effective learning environment as you rewrite your sexual narrative. You can even start integrating these skills immediately while reading to help you learn the content more effectively, such as in moments when you notice you're not feeling fully present.

Another time to use somatic practices is when you feel emotionally hijacked by something you read or any unpleasant experience you have. Using them in this way will help you achieve your sexual wellness goals quicker and easier than if you didn't practice them. Many people feel a natural inclination to push through or ignore uncomfortable feelings; in some scenarios, that can be helpful or adaptive. I invite you to determine when to do that versus when it would be best to try regulating your nervous system with somatic practices. Avoid pushing through or tolerating discomfort when trying to rewire your brain for arousal and pleasure. Further along in the book, we'll explore how to gradually push up against the edges of discomfort to grow and heal, but for now, you'll want to feel well-practiced with these somatic exercises first.

You can use somatic practices when dealing with difficult conversations, managing stressful situations, or if you have a challenge reading the topics in this book. Somatic practices are also excellent even when you feel generally good and want to improve your mood.

While these practices can be very effective in various situations, when you first start using them, they are most helpful with emotions or situations that are at a mild or low-moderate level of distress. Practically speaking, I suggest using them in scenarios that would upset you at a level of three (*maybe* four) out of ten, where ten is the worst thing you could experience.

For me, this is like when I stub my toe hard enough to stop walking and groaning my favorite swear word but not painful enough that I seriously worry it's broken. For an example related to emotions, it might be when my partner is grumpy and snaps at me but apologizes shortly after. You might have different distress levels and emotional reactions to scenarios like that, so listen to your body's own assessment around what elicits mild or low-moderate distress levels.

Although these somatics skills can help lowering levels of momentary distress, only regular exposure to these practices will increase your resilience. Doing so will reduce the impact stressful or upsetting situations have on you. Additionally, the somatic practices can become even more effective with higher levels of distress as you gain more exposure to being embodied and regulating yourself. That's one of the reasons I love somatic work so much—it's a resource that keeps building on itself, creating more resiliency and empowerment as you practice.

Here's a sneak peek of how this portion fits into the overall process of rewiring your brain pathways as it relates to sexual situations.

When anxiety or discomfort arises, the first step is to notice it by paying attention to the present moment and body sensations. Then remember to be kind to yourself because it's not your fault—it's just a learned response from brain pathways paved by constant exposure to unpleasant outcomes. After that, redirect your focus on neutral or pleasant sensations to return you to the present moment and your body while reducing thought spirals that typically keep you in your head. Finally, notice the change in the process to build and strengthen resiliency.

Here's a quick reference for the basic practice you're developing at this point in the book:

1. Create awareness.
2. Build compassion.
3. Redirect focus.
4. Notice the change.

We'll dive more into this in Part 2, but for now I wanted to share with you the trajectory of this process so you can start to see how we create the foundational skill set for increasing arousal and sexual pleasure.

Pleasure Gems

- Somatics (body-based practices) can improve nervous system regulation to decrease the impact of unpleasant emotions, thoughts, and experiences.
- Familiarizing yourself with the practices provided will help you gain control over how you respond to unpleasant experiences instead of being hijacked by them.
- Using somatic practices will enhance your mind-body connection, helping you learn how to overcome emotional and sexual barriers more easily.
- A consistent practice of connecting with your mind-body process will make you feel more present in life and sexual encounters for overall well-being and connection with others.
- You'll gain resiliency and empowerment as you weave somatic awareness and practices into your everyday life and increase your distress tolerance.

Exercises

Quick Wins!

Snapshot and Redirect

Do this as often as you can remember, but aim for two to three times a day.

1. Throughout the day, take a quick Sensation Snapshot to check in with your body.

2. Notice the sensations that are associated with the situation (spend about twenty to thirty seconds doing this). You might only notice unpleasant sensations when you first start practicing this, and that's okay!

3. Next, redirect your attention to a neutral anchor in your body. Notice the sensations in the neutral part of your body (spend at least twenty to thirty seconds with this, or as long as your body needs).

4. If it feels available to you, pay attention to how things in your mind-body shifted from before: Are you feeling less unpleasant? More? Neither but maybe different? If not, that's okay too. There's nothing wrong with what you notice. It's all information; just keep practicing and try not to judge yourself or tell yourself what it means.

Notice Pleasant Sensations

If you don't have time for anything else, the quickest win you can get is by attempting to notice pleasant sensations throughout the day as often as you can.

1. Use your five senses to focus on things in your environment that elicit something pleasant within you (either in your body or mind).

2. Notice what sensations occur in your body as you focus on the pleasant stimuli around you.

Going Deeper

Build Your Own Sensations List

Refer to the Sensations List earlier in the chapter, and as you gain awareness around your own body sensations in response to situations, add them to the list.

When you notice a sensation, ask yourself if it feels pleasant, unpleasant, or neutral. Sometimes, a sensation can feel unpleasant one day and then neutral the next. Although that can feel confusing, it's essential to realize that using somatic awareness is less about getting things right or being the same all the time. Instead, you're mainly focusing on noticing what's happening in the present moment–a core skill for good sex.

Practice "Sensation Snapshot" and "Redirecting to Neutral or Pleasant"

Do each of these three times a day. It will only take about one to two minutes each time you engage in each exercise, but you can also pair them up simultaneously. So that means you're only spending anywhere from six to twelve minutes a day broken up throughout the day to practice somatic regulation—that's totally doable, right?

Do these exercises either when you're feeling neutral (and redirect to pleasant) or when something unpleasant or upsetting occurs (and redirect to neutral or pleasant). *Note: I recommend starting this exercise in moments that feel mostly neutral as you become accustomed to the practice and gain a baseline understanding of your body's sensations when in a mostly neutral state. Then, you can experiment with the intricacies of the exercise when experiencing unpleasant moments.*

If you have difficulty remembering to practice these exercises, write them down where you'll see them regularly (like a sticky note on the fridge). Or set an alarm or notification to remind you to practice.

Some of my clients like to pair these exercises with daily activities. Here are some of their favorites:

- Brushing your teeth
- Going to the bathroom
- Eating food
- Getting into and out of your car
- Drinking water

If you want to engage in the *Going Deeper* exercises throughout the day, but you forget or don't have time, remember that you also have the *Quick Win!* exercise suggestions to use whenever you need.

3

Sexual Mindfulness

One of the most crucial interventions for rewiring your mind and body for better arousal and sexual pleasure is *mindfulness*. Some people love mindfulness and meditation. However, I'm always prepared for the inevitable eye roll and hesitation when I suggest mindfulness to new clients because I know the power it holds and I'm also aware that mindfulness is typically misunderstood. A common complaint I hear from many of my clients is that they hate it because "it doesn't work" for them, or they feel like they're doing it wrong.

If you also struggle, I'd like to offer you a new definition and goal of mindfulness that's helped transform my clients into mindfulness believers.

You might have expectations that mindfulness or meditation is supposed to calm you down or provide peace. And then you try it. Instead of peace, you feel even worse or more distracted than before you started. That's a perfectly typical response because it's what our brains are supposed to do—they're designed to think.

Our brains get distracted for many reasons when we try to sit in quiet meditation or reflection. Contrary to popular belief, it doesn't mean mindfulness or meditation can't be helpful. Instead of aiming for peace, a quiet mind, or to feel calmer, shift those expectations from "goals" to "bonuses." It's great if they happen, but that's not what you're *actually* trying to do.

The *true* goal of mindfulness is to change how we relate to our thoughts. Instead of trying to suppress, change, or do anything else with our thoughts or feelings while meditating, we want to simply notice they exist (without judgment) and then shift back toward the present moment. In my personal meditation practice and for my clients, I suggest noticing neutral or pleasant sensations in the body or around their environment as a helpful anchor or focus.

Your new perspective for mindfulness:

- The goal of mindfulness ≠ *A peaceful, calm, or quiet mind and body.*
- Your new goal for mindfulness = *Changing the way you relate to your thoughts and focusing on neutral or pleasant sensations or environmental experiences.*

By adjusting your expectation of mindfulness from "trying to relax" to "noticing neutral sensations or experiences," your brain and body will learn to relax naturally when it doesn't feel like it *must*. And voilà—mindfulness and meditation become more accessible!

Think about the implications of this regarding sex and arousal. Imagine you want to become more aroused in a fun, pleasure-filled sexual situation, but you keep feeling the pressure of performance anxiety in your head. Telling yourself to focus, spiraling in your thoughts, begging yourself to get turned on so you're not disappointed will ramp up your anxiety, which is the kryptonite of arousal.

Instead of trying to force arousal, imagine what it would be like to focus on neutral sensations or experiences around you, like the feel of the sheets on your body, your deeper breathing, or the sexy music in the background. Your brain reduces its thought spiral and focuses on something that doesn't grip it in anxiety. With time, this can allow your body's natural arousal system to activate pleasantly in many more cases.

With this new goal for mindfulness and a different relationship to have with your thoughts and experiences, you're on the path to becoming connected to your authentic sexual arousal system.

Quick Win! Exercise: Try this concept for a moment. Pause your reading, maybe close your eyes or take a soft gaze, not really trying to see anything. Spend ten to fifteen seconds scanning through your body to check in on how you're feeling or what sensations you notice.

Then, tell yourself to change how you feel. Tell yourself to relax or calm down. Notice what happens as you do that. Does it change? Maybe it does a little. Or maybe you feel more tension arise.

And now, instead of trying to force or change what you're naturally experiencing, direct your attention to notice something neutral in your body: your back against the chair or cushions, the tip of your nose, or maybe your feet on the ground. Spend twenty to thirty seconds focusing on a neutral part of your body. If focusing on your body doesn't feel good right now, then you can focus your thoughts on something neutral like an everyday occurrence, such as washing your hands, pouring water into a glass, or drinking water.

Do you notice a change in your body or mind? Does it feel better, even if it's the slightest? It's okay if not; it might take some time and practice. Plus, it's hard to do this while reading the instructions from a book or trying to remember what to do and practicing at the same time!

Try it out as best as you can for a few days and see if there's a difference between asking your brain and body to calm down and the simple redirection of noticing neutral.

This practice aims to help you embody the differences between forcing relaxation and focusing on neutral as a nervous system regulation technique, which is a building block in rewiring easier arousal and better sex.

Why Mindfulness Improves Everything, Especially Sex

Even though the overall focus of the book is to increase the ease of being sexually aroused and satisfied in ways that align authentically, I promised you that we would start with a more general approach to the content.

At this point in the book, the focus is mainly on creating the best learning environment for having everyday experiences that you find pleasurable and satisfying. We typically learn best when we are present, and that's especially the case when we're learning concepts or behaviors that might conflict with what we previously believed (or were told) to be true, like beliefs about sex.

Using mindfulness helps you on a neurobiological level to regulate (or soothe) your nervous system, allowing you to be more present and improving the impact of the unlearning process.[1] So if you come across belief systems that make you feel bad about yourself, or if you feel uncomfortable with what you're reading or something new you're trying, mindfulness (along with the other skills we're exploring in this part of the book) will be the encouraging and comforting support to keep your momentum going and increasing self-compassion. This will make it easier for you to learn about yourself non-judgmentally, reminding you to be *curious* rather than critical about what's happening to you.

Since mindfulness regulates the nervous system, it also reduces anxiety. When you're more relaxed and present, you can learn new things. You'll also be able to make decisions that align with your present-day values rather than knee-jerk reactions to outdated and harmful belief systems.

Practicing mindfulness outside of the symbolic bedroom helps build the confidence for the skill set that you also need for sex to feel better. The more and more you practice these skills, the easier it will be for your body to remember how to use regulation techniques to soothe anxieties or difficulties related to sex.

Building the confidence to use mindfulness and these other skills in a "low pressure" situation (like in your living room when you have your clothes on and are alone) will also increase your confidence in situations that feel more "high pressured" because you deeply care about the outcome, such as a new sexual experience or communicating with a partner about your arousal needs.

Simple Mindfulness Practices to Try

To follow, I've included some scientifically based practices that have resonated most with my clients so you can try them yourself. You might want to practice each of them a few times in different scenarios to get a full scope of how they might help you (or not).

It could also help to write them down as a "Mindfulness Menu" that you have easy access to. For instance, you could use a sticky note on the cover of this book, a digital note in your phone with a shortcut to it on your home screen, or a reminder written on the mirror so you see it regularly. When we're exposed to these nudges daily it makes change a lot easier. We'll talk more about why this is, along with other helpful habits, in upcoming chapters.

Even though these mindfulness techniques seem simple and straightforward to implement, they are powerful when you find the right ones that work for you. And don't forget the Mindfulness First Aid Kit you can get on my website for free, which you can also use to navigate the book's content or when you feel uncomfortable trying to engage in sexual or romantic experiences.

You can't really go wrong with intentionally using mindfulness. The more you can integrate mindfulness into your regular lifestyle, the more your resiliency grows, and the easier it is to overcome physical obstacles like pain or sexual challenges, and emotional ones like anxiety, depression, and stress.

It's usually pretty difficult to jump right into living mindfully, especially if it's not a skill you've practiced much. Even if mindfulness has been a part of your life for some time, it can still be a challenge. One of the most crucial lessons in this book is that a little goes a long way. This is the case with mindfulness, too. So, let's start slowly.

The following practices are reliable ones I've been using with my clients for over a decade, and maybe you'll like them too. They're not the most mind-blowing suggestions, so be prepared to think, "That's it?! That's the secret??" Yes, some of what you'll find in this book are probably things you've heard before, or they seem so obvious that you might wonder if you're missing something.

As I mentioned, I try to find simple suggestions for a reason: they make it easier to implement them in your daily life, creating the whole model you'll find in this book. If you practice mindfulness (either with my suggestions or others that work for you) in the way I've laid out in the book, you'll see why this has been a crucial part of my clients' successes. The secret to the transformation isn't about each individual exercise or piece of sexual health information. It's about how it all fits together and creates that lasting change. Remember, I intentionally structured this book so that everything builds on itself and facilitates an integrated and cohesive model for sexual wellness and expansion.

Mindfulness Exercise: My Four Faves

Next are my four favorite standard mindfulness practices. Some of my clients like to find guided video or audio on phone apps that focus on the topics mentioned. Alternatively, they record themselves slowly reading the instructions and expanding on them if they need it to be longer. Or if they don't like to record themselves, I will record it for them, which can be really helpful hearing their therapist's or coach's voice, which adds to the regulation they feel because of the comfort they find in our relationship.

I recommend trying these in various scenarios and when experiencing different emotions. Don't give up after the first attempt at any of the exercises described (unless you know that there might be a trauma trigger in them). Sometimes, one of these exercises will feel great on Tuesday and then terrible on Wednesday. The goal of offering multiple options is to help you find the ones that typically work best for you, but you will get a better idea after practicing with them in different ways, multiple times.

You don't need to spend long doing them, either. Sometimes all you need is thirty seconds to get the benefit of mindfulness with enough practice. I was shocked when I realized I could decrease my anxiety and pain without spending ten to twenty minutes a day meditating. Instead of feeling like a failure when I forgot (or, let's be real, when I just didn't *want* to remember) about meditation as a resource for improving my sex life. First, start with one to two minutes trying these out. Notice any shifts in tension, heart rate, or breathing that feel more neutral or pleasant. Give yourself compassion and time; it can take a few attempts before you start to notice anything significant. Celebrate the tiniest shift, even if you only notice one percent less tense, slower breathing, or reduced heart rate—that's a win!

Breathe

Notice how your breath moves through your body. Feel the rising in your lungs and chest. Notice the tickle in the back of your throat or your nostrils as air moves in and out. If focusing on how your body feels is too overwhelming (which happens to many folks), you can notice how your clothes move against your skin as you inhale and exhale. You can also focus on the sound of your breath.

Some people feel more activated or anxious when they focus on their breath. If that's you, try one of the others instead.

Grounding

Notice the sensations of your feet planted on the ground, your tushie on the chair or cushion, or your back against the wall or pillow. This is a beneficial practice if you're feeling anxious, too much in your head, out of your body, or disconnected somehow.

Centering

Imagine a center line or core within your body or just in front of your body. Imagine that it lengthens your spine and opens up your body in a supportive and calming way. Notice the sensations as you imagine this.

If you're feeling disconnected from your values, goals, or sense of who you are, this can be useful for reconnecting with your center core and purpose.

Movement

Engage in a movement that your body says "yes" to. It can be a slow walk, focusing on feeling your weight transfer from side to side. You can wiggle your body however it wants to in that moment. You can shake out your arms or legs (or both), do push-ups, dance, or spin in a circle. Whatever you choose, do it and focus on the sensations of each movement as best as you can.

Using movement as a mindfulness practice like this can be helpful when you're feeling an excess of unpleasant or disconnecting energy (as opposed to pleasant and embodied energy).

Mindfulness Exercise: Body Scanwich

The Body Scanwich is a one-to-two-minute mindfulness practice that I teach all my clients at the beginning of our work. I created it to help them (and now, you) experience and understand the rewiring process that happens while doing this work.

It starts with a twenty-to-thirty-second body scan, followed by a twenty-to-thirty-second mindfulness practice, and wraps up with another twenty-to-thirty-second body scan. It's a body scan sandwich . . . a Body Scanwich, get it? LOL . . . it's the small things.

This tool is crucial to facilitate change neurobiologically or when dealing with difficult emotions or experiences. Regardless of whether you use the Body Scanwich for stress from work, anxieties about sex, or if someone cuts you off on the highway, practicing it as often as you can and in as many scenarios as you can will be incredibly beneficial.

The first body scan is meant to help you notice what's happening in your body first in order to develop a baseline. Try to avoid judgment or an impulse to actively change anything that you notice as you do the scan. The goal in this first step is to simply take a snapshot of your body's sensations and feelings: Are you tense in one area, more relaxed and grounded in another? Are you feeling anxious all over? Do you have trouble feeling or noticing anything? These are totally normal to experience. Don't comment on what you notice; don't try to change anything. Your only goal is to observe. You'll use the information collected from this first body scan at the end of the Body Scanwich. Remember, this practice (and the whole book) is designed to help you rewire your brain based on the neuroscience of creating change.

In the next step of this exercise, use a mindfulness practice that you enjoy for twenty to thirty seconds. You can use one of the suggestions in this book or anything else that inspires you to focus on the present moment in a neutral or pleasant way.

Finally, you'll end the Body Scanwich with a second body scan. You'll do it just like you did the first time, except this time, the focus will be on sensing any change when comparing how your body is now to how it was before the mindfulness practice. Notice if you're less tense in some areas than you were before. Or maybe you're more tense, and that's okay too. Avoid judging what you notice; it doesn't mean you did anything wrong.

Sometimes, when we get present and focused on our bodies, we realize how bad things feel or how hard things are right now. If this happens to you, avoid beating yourself up, and don't give up on the practice. Try it a few more times in different scenarios. If it still happens, it could indicate that you might need more experienced insight. Reach out, and we can help you find solutions.

If you dissociate during this practice (meaning you feel floaty, disembodied, or completely disconnected from yourself or even reality), having a professional trained in somatically focused trauma treatment help you will be significantly beneficial because it might indicate that you're experiencing a trauma response (even if you have no identifiable traumas in your past). In that case, I love supporting clients through this, too.

Mindfulness Tips

Remember, practicing compassion when you engage in any mindfulness exercise is extremely important. Try to release how you think it should look or feel. You don't have to find any meaning or stories about what you experience—that will take you out of the present moment.

These practices are designed to be done in a short period of time. You don't need to spend ten to twenty minutes meditating daily to get the beneficial effects of these nervous system regulation techniques. My clients are often surprised when I suggest trying one to five minutes, one to three times daily. If you find it isn't easy to do that, see what it's like to try it for only twenty seconds, as often as you can, but at least daily.

Notice what happens in your body as you practice these effective mindfulness tools. If it's hard for you to focus inward on your body, you can notice any general shift or change in your mood or feelings. *The goal is to seek neutral experiences.*

It's normal if you can't stay in the present moment for more than a few seconds. Your brain is designed to think, seek solutions, and otherwise get distracted.

Your most fundamental tool in rewiring your brain for arousal and pleasure is to return to the present moment when you notice when you're distracted, feeling something unpleasant, or disconnected from your body. It's as simple as that—simple but not easy. You'll learn more about how to apply this to sexual situations in Part 2.

Starting with any of these practices immediately and as you read through the book will move your progress forward more powerfully than you might realize. With time, you'll start to notice the effects of your efforts when you can stop negative thought spirals more easily, or when you find pleasure in sensual moments when you previously felt discomfort. Eventually, it will be exciting when you feel a little more confident in expressing your sexual preferences without feeling guilty—even if that means you aren't interested in sexual play at that moment.

When to Use Mindfulness for Building Sexual Resiliency

Since we're focusing on practicing these tools before introducing sexual context, I recommend using mindfulness or somatic practices that resonated if you find yourself in any of the following scenarios to build "muscle memory." Later, we'll bring these concepts into your sex life.

- Any time you're feeling unpleasant emotions or sensations in your body.
- If you start to feel unpleasant, negative, or hard on yourself or you notice shame or guilt creeping in as you read, pause and try one of the practices in this chapter, then return to the book.
- If you notice that you have set the book down for a while, promising to return later, but keep making excuses and don't return to it. Or you

experience unpleasant feelings or hear negative self-talk when you think about returning to the book, instead of beating yourself up about the avoidance dance you're in, try mindfulness practices. Then see how it would feel to just read one page of the book. Check in with your body after you read a page and then try another mindfulness exercise. Then try reading two pages before needing to engage in mindfulness again. Continue this practice until it feels at least neutral, and you're not engaging in critical self-talk or experiencing overwhelming unpleasantness.

- Before, during, or after a difficult conversation with someone.
- Even when you're not feeling particularly unpleasant, set an alarm to practice them. This is an extremely helpful way to feel the impact of mindfulness in different ways.

Remember, if you have difficulty with mindfulness practices, know it's completely normal. Give yourself permission to fumble with them. The goal is to simply notice what's happening as you try them; they will become easier with time.

If you're still having trouble, reach out because helping people find mindfulness practices that work for them is something I love doing. Sometimes, a person needs an individually tailored plan on how to navigate mindfulness practices because it's not a one-size-fits-all approach, especially when it relates to something as complex as dealing with sexual challenges.

Pleasure Gems

- A new perspective that can make mindfulness and meditation a lot easier: the goal is to change the way you relate to your thoughts and experiences instead of forcing relaxation.
- Mindfulness is a tool to facilitate lasting change because it helps with paving new belief systems, particularly around sex.

- Mindfulness regulates our nervous system which makes it easier to learn new concepts or behaviors, even when the topic might feel emotionally challenging.
- Utilize mindfulness practices from this chapter that you can use daily without them feeling like chores.

Exercises

Quick Wins!

Forcing Relaxation vs. Noticing Neutral

Notice the difference between trying to force yourself to calm down or relax and identifying neutral or pleasant sensations. Then notice the impact these two different experiences have on your body and mood.

For a free download of this and other mindfulness resources, head over to my website: www.cassardcenter.com/freebies.

Mindfulness Practice Quickie

Try one of the mindfulness practices for twenty to thirty seconds one to three times daily.

Going Deeper

Create a Mindfulness Menu

- Choose a few of the exercises in this chapter.
- Practice with them one to three minutes, three times a day.
- Add the ones you like the most to your Mindfulness Menu.
- Put the menu somewhere you'll see it regularly.

4

Cultivating a Pleasure-Based Mindset

Your mindset (how you view your situation and engage in problem-solving) is crucial to shifting to a more comfortable and satisfying sex and romantic life, no matter how you feel about sex. This chapter will explain your new powerful tool for rewiring brain pathways for authentic arousal and pleasure.

The popular concept folks call "mindset work" involves using a growth mindset for personal development. A "growth mindset," first coined by psychologist Dr. Carol Dweck, is the belief that abilities and intelligence can improve through dedication and effort.[1]

Someone with a *growth mindset* sees challenges as opportunities and criticism as feedback. They actively seek support and knowledge from others with more experience and are interested in finding effective strategies for a better life. Developing this mindset enhances resilience and motivation, which are critical contributors to success in making positive changes in their lives.

Here are some thoughts or beliefs my clients have shared that reflect a growth mindset as they've progressed in their sexual journeys:

- "I've had challenges with sex, but I'm learning new ways to relate to my sexual experience and my mind-body connection."

- "An obstacle around my sexual life is an opportunity to learn more about myself and grow."
- "My sexual response doesn't have to meet anyone else's expectations or definitions. I can be aroused by whatever feels good to me."

The opposite of a growth mindset is a "static" or "fixed mindset." Someone with a *fixed mindset* believes that intelligence and abilities are innate and unchangeable. They are often significantly discouraged by minor setbacks and do not value using external resources to improve their skills or intelligence.

Below are some thoughts or beliefs within a fixed mindset that clients have shared when they started their work with me:

- "The only way I get aroused or feel sexually pleased or intimately connected is with penis-in-vagina (PIV) sex. I can't change that."
- "I've always gotten off this way, and nothing else will ever work either."
- "That's just the way guys/gals/people are."
- "Even though I get aroused by something my family/culture/religion thinks is taboo, I have to keep suppressing my authentic desires no matter how much it hurts or how much shame I feel."

Hopefully, you can see the difference between growth and fixed mindsets. If you find yourself in the fixed mindset group, don't worry—there's nothing wrong with you. You're reading this book because you want to improve your sex life, and that's a remarkable first step. Soon enough, you'll learn to uncover fixed mindsets and belief systems that may keep you stuck. For now, be compassionate with yourself and know that mindset work can help you transform.

Changing deeply rooted beliefs or thoughts might seem impossible, especially if they're tied to your upbringing or core values. That's okay. Just stay curious and open-minded as we go.

Mindset work can significantly impact how you feel and think about yourself, helping you engage with your body and partners in authentic and delicious ways. A key goal is *finding alignment*: where your inner thoughts, desires, and beliefs match your outer actions and interactions. A growth mindset is a powerful tool for achieving this alignment.

Empowered Belief Systems Build Sexual Resilience

Mindset work is a powerful tool, but it needs to be approached through a trauma-informed lens that acknowledges the body's experience and recognizes the very real barriers created by trauma, oppression, and systemic injustice. I'm not exaggerating when I say that somatic and trauma-informed mindset coaching makes up about a third of my work with both psychotherapy and coaching clients. Many of them have been so immersed in the oppressive narratives for so long that they don't even realize how deeply those influences have shaped every aspect of their lives. I spend a lot less time teaching the "technical skills" of building sexual arousal and relationship techniques than most people think I do.

Just like those clients, you've probably encountered similar, defeating messages around sex, so you need to adopt a mindset that empowers and assists you to utilize your existing resources, such as your thoughts, body sensations, and current skills (even if unrelated to sex). By doing this, you're not starting from square one. Instead, you're learning to apply what you already know to newer concepts around sex and arousal, leading to more confidence-boosting momentum.

Here's an amazing example of the kind of shifts this mindset approach can provide.

Case Study: Rae (she/them)

One of my clients, Rae, was having difficulty sleeping, and it was impacting everything, from work to health to sexual wellness. She got a smartwatch to track her sleeping patterns. After wearing it for thirty days, Rae learned she wasn't getting enough deep sleep. Only about 15 percent of her sleep was in deep sleep (scientists say we should aim for 20–25 percent).[2] Since we had been starting to talk about somatic mindset work (which Rae wasn't entirely buying into), this was an opportunity for her to gain tangible feedback to help her determine if this kind of mindset work could benefit her. We planned a simple test: somatically incorporate mindset sleep affirmations for a week and see what happens.

Rae identified a sleep affirmation (an encouraging phrase about getting deep sleep) and paired it with the somatic practice of noticing where in her body she felt relaxation. She committed to doing this for about three to five minutes before sleeping. We were both shocked when she realized she didn't even need the whole week to see the impact of the change—after two nights, Rae was hitting the benchmark for deeper sleep! It continued, improving over time. Rae became a believer. We used this new belief system (which Rae decided was "By focusing on pleasant sensations, I can influence how my body operates!"). Rae applied this affirmation to sex, along with somatic practices, to decrease performance anxiety during sex. It helped tremendously.

As it relates directly to sexual pain, anxiety, or intimacy barriers, my clients have used the following encouraging phrases while also noticing pleasant or neutral sensations in their bodies that arise when they say them (out loud or in their heads):

- "Physical or intimate connection does not have to lead to sex."
- "Pain (or anxiety) might make me feel uncomfortable, but I am in charge of my mind and body."
- "I am loved no matter the kind of sex I can (or want to) have."
- "My worth is not dependent upon how my body performs."
- "My vagina (or anus) is relaxed, open, and willing to receive penetration."

These phrases on their own are considered "positive affirmations," and I can almost hear the eye roll that usually comes with the idea of using positive affirmations for improving sex. I totally get it. I felt the same way, too. This is why I don't prescribe just *any* positive affirmations to mindset work. Effective positive affirmations incorporate more than just saying a nice phrase. In my programs, I get more detailed with creating effective affirmations, but the basic steps are twofold: choose something you believe now *and* for the future, and pair it with a somatic practice so you can feel the impact of the desired outcome imprinted into your body via sensations. You'll explore how to do the latter step in a later chapter.

Mindset Beliefs for Rewriting Your Sexual Narrative

The next step in working toward rewriting your narrative is to establish some general sexual mindset beliefs supporting sexual resilience. I've provided some Sexually Empowered Sex Mindset Beliefs in this section that I'd like you to consider and determine if they align with you.

If they don't align, I invite you to explore why that might be the case. It could be because it just doesn't fit, and that's totally fine—you get to choose what feels suitable for you.

One or more of the Mindset Beliefs might not fit because some deeply wired belief systems need more love and attention before you decide to reconsider them. As discussed in the first few chapters, belief systems are sometimes created because they protect you from something, or it's all you've known. So, I invite you to find gratitude for the outdated belief system that tried to protect you or connect you to the people you care about, however unhelpful it may be now. Since conflict around sex arises when our internal experiences (desires) and our external experiences (behaviors) are not aligned, that's when we could examine belief systems that are no longer serving us.

For example, at one point in your life, you knew without a doubt that a parent, caregiver, or other adult was necessary for your survival: you needed them to prepare food, keep you warm and healthy, and help you walk. That belief was the absolute truth in your life for some time, and your brain was wired to believe it without a doubt. Then, one day, you started to have experiences where you didn't always have to rely on someone else. Eventually, you didn't need them anymore (although I'm sure I'm not alone in wanting someone else to prepare my food daily).

Now, can you imagine the difficulties you would face if, as an adult, you still held onto the belief that someone else needs to do these things for you? Holding on to beliefs that were created when you needed them becomes a problem if you continue to believe them beyond their expiration dates.

There might be some beliefs you want to release and others you don't because they are woven into larger cultural or religious belief systems. However, you might still have issues with sex due to some belief systems, and you're not sure how to change them without tearing the fabric of your core belief system wide open.

Let's look at how mindset work can help with something like that.

Case Study: Bethany (she/her) and John (he/him)

Bethany's and John's challenges reflected an issue I regularly see in my practice. They both explained that they are loyally committed to their religion, which believes that a certain kind of sex (penis-in-vagina or PIV) between two people should be reserved for after marriage. They didn't attempt to engage in it until their honeymoon, which didn't work out—she felt pain upon penetration, and he felt so anxious that he was unable to maintain an erection. They continued to run up against the same barriers for the first several months of their marriage. Bethany and John were confused and frustrated. They worried this meant something bad about their marriage, mainly because they engaged in other kinds of sex before their marriage without problems.

However, I explained to them the concept of conflicting belief systems. In their case, the outdated belief system for their relationship was "no sex before marriage." Even though that belief was no longer necessary, their bodies didn't suddenly release the tension and importance that came with "no sex before marriage." Their bodies didn't know that they had signed a marriage certificate indicating it was acceptable to have PIV sex now. It was too deeply woven into their brain pathways as an undeniable "truth" that "sex" was "unsafe" or "a threat" to their belief system.

Their desire for a new belief system ("We're married now, we can have all the sex we want") wasn't reaching their mind-body connection. By understanding that they can rewire their brains with practical steps, mindfulness, and somatic interventions, they could teach their bodies that engaging in penetration is "safe" now because that former belief system had become outdated (for them). They still held onto their core religious and cultural belief systems and rewired new ones that aligned with the parts of themselves that they still valued.

Mindset work can be mighty when you are willing to explore your belief systems in a non-critical and objective way. I'm not asking you to uproot everything you believe in entirely. Instead, I'm inviting you to review all belief systems that might be impacting your sexual well-being so you can start to identify which are working, which aren't, and which you might be able to adjust slightly so that you can live in alignment and have better and better sex.

The following Sexually Empowered Mindset Beliefs can support a foundational beginning to a healthy sexual response system and overall sexual well-being, so I invite you to keep them at the top of your mind as you continue to read through the book.

Additionally, if some (or all) of them are new to you, I hope you're open to creating new pathways for more adaptive belief systems by using the skills we've already discussed as you read the following mindset beliefs.

To do this, notice the pleasant sensations in your body as you reflect on them. Here's a bonus tip to take the internal learning even further: If you notice a "lightbulb moment," an experience that feels like an epiphany, or anything else that feels inspiring, notice where in your body the new belief feels "true." What sensations do you also notice in that part of your body? Lightness, energy, tingling, movement, opening, or expansion are common responses to something like this, but yours might differ. There's no judgment if you don't feel something like that, though.

Sexually Empowered Mindset Belief #1: Your Most Influential Sexual Organ Is Your Brain

Sexual health education is only one part of the equation. All the knowledge about sexual wellness, sexual skills, and arousal won't matter if you don't also have the tools to actually use those skills effectively.

Case in point: A client started working with me because he was distressed about his marriage and sex life. He had difficulty getting and maintaining an erection when he wanted to, even with the use of supportive medication like Viagra® or Cialis®. Taking those medications had helped him previously, but then they started to become hit or miss. After a lengthy exploration into the dynamic of his marriage and how he felt about the pressures of performing, he realized that his thoughts and belief systems were the true boner-killers.

Embracing the idea that using your brain is just as important as using your genitals for sexual arousal and satisfaction is a crucial concept in moving forward.

Sexually Empowered Mindset Belief #2: Understanding How to Make Your Brain Work for You Rather than Against You Is Half the Battle

This mindset belief is a sister to the first one. You now know from previous chapters that a neurobiological process helps create learned responses and changes on a cellular level. Hopefully, you've been practicing the exercises to understand this in your mind and experience it in your body.

Owning this belief means that you are taking control of your sexual arousal and pleasure however you can. You can unlearn outdated beliefs and rewire your brain for a new narrative. With that knowledge and power, you recognize that you're not at the mercy of what others tell you is "normal." Actively using your brain as an ally will optimize your growth and resilience.

Sexually Empowered Mindset Belief #3: Focus on the Journey, Not the Destination

This belief is so essential for most things in life, but especially for sex. Many people think that the point or goal of sex is to end in orgasm. While that may be a fantastic bonus, it can cause issues if it's always the focus. That's because it makes the act of sex goal-oriented instead of pleasure-based. Being "pleasure-based" means engaging in sexual play simply for the pleasure of the whole experience.

By learning to focus on the process (the journey), you build the skills to improve your experience. As a result, the destination is usually a lot more satisfying.

Sexually Empowered Mindset Belief #4: Cultivate Curiosity and Kindness, Being as Objective as You Can

The previous chapters introduced you to the concept of curiosity. Using your curiosity to guide your experiences (instead of a judge and jury) reduces emotional and physical tension, increases compassion, and unlocks possibilities for more enjoyable experiences.

This belief helps with busting perfectionism by encouraging the idea that you might never feel completely ready or prepared to (gently) push out of your comfort zone. Start before you feel ready and know there are no "failures," only learning opportunities. Everything about this book is to encourage you to be in the process of always learning. Think of yourself as a compassionate and sexy scientist; you're collecting data about what felt good or could shift so that you might enjoy it more next time. There's no right or wrong.

A simple but effective phrase you can use is "Isn't that interesting?" whenever you encounter something you don't enjoy or feel tension. Understand which information can be gathered from the experience, notice how your body responds to it, and use that to determine how you would like it to adjust the next time you try. Utilizing this belief system and process can elicit more compassion for yourself, keeping you from spiraling into self-criticism or shame. This contrasts with "I failed," "I'm a disappointment," "That was bad," or any other judgmental thoughts that arise when faced with sexual challenges.

Practically, this might look like attempting to engage in sexual play with yourself or a partner, and despite wanting to be aroused, after some time, you find that you become distracted and eventually stop. Instead of asking, "What's wrong with me?," "How could I fail again at this?" with this new belief, you would cultivate curiosity and explore what was going on that distracted you. You might reflect on what you were feeling before, during, or after the sexual scenario. You could also think about what else was going on in the day that might influence your state of mind. This helps interrupt the guilt-shame spiral that often comes with sexual challenges.

Ultimately, your goal is to learn more about yourself, not achieve a particular outcome based on success or failure.

Sexually Empowered Mindset Belief #5: Regulated Perseverance Creates Sexual Resilience

We'll get into the details about sexual resilience in Part 2, but the main idea I want to bring to your attention right now is the power of regulated perseverance in mindset work. Contrary to what we've been told, most sex (especially "good sex") doesn't just happen magically or naturally. Sex and arousal are aspects of life that require practice, dedication, and intention without giving up or assuming something is wrong when sex doesn't happen as you might expect or hope. Sex doesn't always go as planned; arousal may dip and fade during parts of your life, or you might not see eye to eye with your partner sometimes, and this can be a wet blanket for your arousal. Increasing your capacity for regulated perseverance is essential for developing muscle memory and recovering from difficulties, feelings of failure, or rejection.

A business study researching the importance of perseverance and consistency in entrepreneurial success identified that the more grit a person has, the more successful they are.[3] Even though we're not talking about boardrooms and strategic analyses in this book, sex and relationships can learn a lot from successful businesses in many more ways than you might realize. To bring it closer to our focus here, in another study, researchers found that resilience, persistence, and a positive outlook on achieving goals within a romantic or intimate relationship reflected increased well-being individually and within the partnership.[4]

Grit, perseverance, and persistence can sometimes be considered a little too extreme in the sense that folks will "push through" or simply "tolerate." That's not what we're going for here. Using the skills and awareness we discussed with mindfulness and somatics regarding "nervous system regulation," you'll build sexual resilience through regulated and embodied perseverance. To do this, it will be essential to pay attention to your body's cues that tell you the difference between bracing and pushing gently up against the edges of discomfort while feeling grounded or encouraged by the process. This can be really hard to distinguish, especially if you're a people-pleaser, perfectionist, or caregiver, or you've had trauma in the past. If you keep running into this barrier of uncertainty about how you're building sexual resiliency, that's where a somatic sex therapist can support you!

Mindset Interventions for Rewriting Your Sexual Narrative

Mindset work like this is instrumental for those of us who are "in our heads" a lot and like to have mental strategies to interrupt brain spirals or out-of-control thinking. Many of the following tools are informed by evidence-based cognitive behavioral strategies and include my somatic spin on them for more effective implementation into your sexual wellness.

Don't forget the power of using them in everyday life too—that will help you integrate them even further.

Adopt the Power of Pivoting

A favorite moment in the *Friends* sitcom is when Ross, Chandler, and Rachel attempt to move a couch up several floors of stairs. Ross hilariously screams "Pivot!" as they try to get it to fit through the turns without much success. I'm also offering "pivot" to you, but in a way that I think will work much better than it did for Ross. For our purposes, pivoting redirects focus or effort when you notice resistance to something and seek more inviting alternatives.

Practically speaking, this might look like one of the following examples:

- You attempt to engage in a specific style of masturbating or a sexual position that has somehow lost its effect or is not feeling as pleasing as you would like it to and shift to another style or position.

- When you (or your partner) don't have the kind of erection (penile or clitoral) desired, and you find it difficult to get out of your head, instead of getting frustrated and stopping, you choose something else that feels pleasurable.

In sexual experiences, if you don't pivot because feelings are tense or options seem limited (and you would prefer to continue), it can lead to further disappointment, guilt, or frustration, among other unpleasant feelings. On a neurobiological level, ending the sexual play or experience instead of pivoting can reinforce challenging feelings, thoughts, or experiences. It strengthens the brain's pathway that "sex" equates to unpleasant associations. But always remember, you or your partner(s) always have the right to stop anything at any time without consequence.

When you pivot, you give yourself a chance to rewire your brain for more growth and change that aligns with your larger goals of a satisfying sex life. Paired with the other techniques in this book, you're building a growth mindset as you become a scientist and engage in problem-solving instead of defeat when confronted with obstacles.

Develop Growth-Oriented Environments

A "growth-oriented environment" is more than just a fancy term; it's a powerful concept that can empower you by surrounding yourself with like-minded individuals and lifestyles that foster a growth mindset. While success is possible without this environment, being around others who use solution-focused and empowering language amplifies your efforts.

I've seen and experienced the power of community in achieving goals across various areas, from business to mental health to sexual satisfaction. Since the pandemic started in 2020, I've offered a virtual support group for people struggling with sexual challenges like pain, low libido, and orgasm difficulties.

Research shows that support groups and community involvement significantly enhance wellness and help overcome sexual issues, particularly sexual pain.[5] Hearing success stories from others with a growth mindset can be incredibly inspiring, reminding you of lessons learned and strategies to try. Being part of a community with shared goals and similar journeys ignites motivation, helping you maintain momentum and accountability.

Some clients find support in online communities like Facebook groups or Reddit. However, be cautious about relying solely on these groups, as they often contain posts reflecting fixed mindsets, focusing on problems rather than solutions, which can subconsciously hinder growth.

Surrounding yourself with thoughts, experiences, and people that align with your values and goals makes the process easier and helps you feel supported, especially during challenging times.

Redefine "Success" by Celebrating (Seemingly) Small Wins

Many people struggle with reaching their sexual goals because they have narrow expectations influenced by media and porn. They see sex as a "pass/fail" activity, focusing on outcomes like orgasm or maintaining an erection. However, healthy and satisfying sex is more about the journey than the destination. This is where a pleasure-focused mindset comes into play.

Redefining "successful" sexual experiences helps create easier arousal, more pleasure, and a satisfying sex life. Instead of viewing them as "success vs. failure," think about them from a pleasure-oriented perspective. Consider these questions:

- Did I engage mindfully with myself or my partner(s)?
- Did I ask for what I needed to feel comfortable and focus on pleasure?
- Was I kind to myself when I felt anxious or distracted?

- Did I seek pleasure instead of criticism?
- Did I connect with my partner(s)?
- Did I engage in sex how I wanted, not just what was expected?

If the answer to these questions is "no," use kind thoughts and curiosity to understand why and how to adjust next time. Redefining success liberates you from rigid sexual standards and allows you to celebrate small wins, reinforcing new, healthier pathways.

You get to decide what good sex looks like to you. You can change your definitions as often as you want or even have multiple meanings of "good sex," depending on if you're having solo sex, who you're having sex with, or what kind of mood you're in.

Shifting your mindset from a singular outcome like orgasm to multiple moments of enjoyment creates more opportunities for satisfying experiences. Celebrating these small wins helps challenge outdated beliefs. It fosters a sense of control and empowerment, which is crucial for behavior change and improved health.[6]

As you gain knowledge about yourself, sex, arousal, and your partner(s), you'll acquire skills and confidence, reducing anxiety. The book *Slight Edge* explains that reducing anxiety comes from increasing mastery.[7] While we're not aiming for "mastery" over sex, think of it as mastering your sex life in a way that aligns with your new definitions of success—liberating, embodied, and exciting.

Imprint the Shifts

Engaging in change around how you relate to arousal, sex, and pleasure requires a lot more than just telling yourself to change. As you've learned, body sensations can deepen the impact of the shifts you're making, creating "imprints" of liberating narratives via new neural pathways.

Let's try a quick exercise to experience this:

1. First, think about a belief that seems to get in the way of your authentic sexual expression (this is called a Limiting Belief).
2. Take a Sensation Snapshot for twenty seconds and notice how your body reacts.
3. Then, shift to a new belief related to the Limiting Belief but one that feels liberating or empowering (this is your Empowered Belief).
4. Focus on that belief for twenty–thirty seconds.
5. Take another Sensation Snapshot and observe any changes in your body.

Did you notice a difference? Even a tiny shift toward more neutral or pleasant is okay. If you didn't feel a change, that's fine too; you might still be learning your body's language, which takes time.

The sensations that arise when thinking about your Empowered Beliefs are starting to create new pathways in your brain and body. By identifying Limiting Beliefs and questioning their importance, you open the possibility for new, more robust pathways. Reinforce these Empowered Beliefs by bringing them to the forefront of your mind and aligning your thoughts and behaviors with them.

As you have new thoughts or engage in new behaviors, deepen the learning by focusing on the neutral or pleasant sensations as they occur. This exposure helps Empowered Beliefs become stronger while Limiting Beliefs lose their grip and increases your resilience.

Troubleshooting Mindset Transformations

Developing a sexual growth mindset will likely result in eventually facing obstacles like perfectionism, self-doubt, or fear of failure. These challenges signify crucial milestones in your growth journey, signaling you're pushing boundaries and evolving. Recognize these obstacles as natural defense mechanisms your brain uses to maintain the status quo. Reframing resistance as "important work" can help release associated shame and keep momentum through the process.

Perfectionism often manifests as a barrier. Fear of failure or reluctance to try new things can hint at its influence even if you don't identify as a perfectionist. Think of perfectionism as an outdated belief system trying to protect you from failure. To transform perfectionism, acknowledge its role, appreciate its intention, and remind yourself that you have new tools to redefine and achieve success. Then, imprint the shift in your body.

Give yourself permission to make mistakes, be imperfect, and experience discomfort. Many clients fear awkwardness in exploring new sexual experiences, but normalizing this discomfort often brings relief.

Finally, not knowing what you want sexually beyond basic ideas or "norms" influenced by a sex-negative culture is a common barrier. This experience often creates feelings of sexual inadequacy. People need a safe, relatable model to explore their pleasure practices. I developed the Arousal Architecture®, a framework for exploring pleasure practices, detailed in Part 3 to address this.

Starting from a place of "not knowing" is fertile ground for exploration. It's like a blank canvas waiting for you to paint on. The tools we've discussed and what's ahead will help you choose your colors and create your unique, sexually satisfying masterpiece.

When Mindset Work Isn't Enough

If, despite all your efforts to implement the techniques and structures we've discussed, you still feel stuck or want your process to move along quicker, you might need more than just a growth mindset to navigate through. Somatic psychotherapy, sex therapy, or trauma therapy can help you identify deeper blockages and work through them in a safe, contained, and supportive space.

It's necessary to work with a specialist who has been trained or certified in trauma-informed care or therapy because topics around sex can be so steeped in shame that talking about them without the right kind of container could continue to reinforce harmful belief systems. Plenty of resources are at the back of the book to help you locate support.

Pleasure Gems

- A growth mindset is one of the most influential tools for optimizing and improving sexual experiences and personal development.
- You gained new perspectives and ways to interact with your thoughts, feelings, and beliefs around arousal, pleasure, and sex to help you with a tangible path forward on rewriting your sexual narratives and rewiring brain pathways.
- There are a variety of mindset interventions available to you to support your new sexual narrative including pivoting, redefining success, finding community, and imprinting.
- Resistance, perfectionism, or self-doubt are common experiences when trying to make significant change. Keep trucking with regulated perseverance to improve confidence.

Exercises

Quick Win!

Reframe an Automatic Thought with a Compassionate Script
Most people can't shift from believing one thing to something new without a few steps in between. One of those steps is making space for the feelings

or emotions that arise when exploring the conflict between your current, deeply wired beliefs and the desire for different, new, and sometimes opposite beliefs.

Ignoring the feelings that come up around sex, arousal, intimacy, or your relationships will likely cause problems later, and you'll just have to deal with them then. At that point, the feelings have probably festered into something that feels even bigger to overcome and has probably caused havoc over time, whether you've noticed or not.

Use the following script when you notice critical self-talk arising: "Of course, I would [do this thing, think this way, feel like this], it's rooted in past patterns. It makes sense I feel this way." Imprint the shift in your body to make it more impactful.

Going Deeper

Identify Limiting Beliefs

Take a moment to jot down any Limiting Beliefs you hold about sex that you want to challenge. These beliefs might be thoughts about sex or arousal that you know aren't aligned with what you genuinely desire but find difficult to let go of. For example, you might write, "Sexual arousal should always come naturally if I'm truly attracted to my partner."

As you go about your day or week, stay alert for any other Limiting Beliefs that come to mind. The more you consciously bring these thoughts about sex into your awareness, the more control you'll gain over changing them if you discover they no longer serve you.

Identify Empowered Beliefs

Jot down Empowered Beliefs you would like to incorporate into your authentic experience. Knowing what you're working toward is powerful, but writing it down deepens the process of rewiring your sexual narrative.

You could use the Limiting Beliefs you identified to stimulate ideas for what you wish to believe instead.

Imprint New Beliefs in Your Body

Choose an Empowered Belief to "try on" daily for several days. Here's how you'll try it on:

1. As you think about your Empowered Belief, imagine for two minutes that you believe it deep in your bones. Notice the sensations that come up as you do that.
2. To intensify the experience:
   - Imagine scenes that would occur as you fully embrace this belief.
   - Think about how you would talk differently, act differently, or how your life would be different.
3. Continue to notice the sensations as you let your imagination run wild with this Empowered Belief as your reality.

Try this daily for as long as you can or choose a set number of days. I encourage my clients to try a sixty-six-day challenge. Research has shown that sixty-six days is the average amount of time it takes participants to form a new habit.[8] If sixty-six days seems like a lot, choose something that feels doable.

I tried this challenge using the affirmation, "My power is available for me to access whenever I need it," while brushing my teeth. I had unbelievable results!

If you want to download an editable sixty-six-day calendar I created for this, head over to my website: www.cassardcenter.com/freebies.

PART 2

LET'S GET GEEKY ABOUT YOUR AROUSAL POTENTIAL

Many people seek my help after trying various methods such as prescription medications, injections, or hormone therapy to solve their sexual problems, not realizing they have untapped tools within themselves. By combining brain, body, and energy with sexual science and pleasure, I help clients find solutions that don't always require medical intervention. They learn that healthy, pleasure-based sex education, a clear road map, and somatic guidance can transform their sexual lives.

Sexual challenges like low libido, performance anxiety, painful sex, or erectile variability are best treated by addressing three core areas:

- *Medical or Physical*: Issues with organs, tissues, or muscles, for instance.
- *Relational or Interpersonal*: Problems arising from relationship conflicts or intimacy barriers.
- *Intrapersonal*: Psychological challenges like anxiety, guilt, or shame.

Research shows that a multidisciplinary treatment team is the most effective for most sexual issues.[1] This team might include medical doctors (urologists or gynecologists), physical therapists, and psychotherapists skilled in sexual science and sex therapy. Ensure any professional you consult has specific training in sexual science, sex therapy, or a sex-positive approach to avoid accidental shaming.

A comprehensive, trauma-informed approach involves incorporating your whole being and relationships to access lasting change. A bio-psycho-social-cultural model addresses medical, emotional, relational, and societal aspects of your experience, unlocking lifelong sexual confidence and empowerment.

I joke with my clients that they start working with me to improve sex, but they stay for the all-encompassing life transformation. Using the model and techniques in this book has helped my clients achieve well-deserved promotions, weed out toxic friendships, deepen connections with their families, and find more meaningful purpose in their lives.

Ready for Empowerment in Sex and Beyond?

In Part 2, you'll gain knowledge and skills to understand how your brain, body, and energy work together for more pleasurable sex. This information is as essential as understanding how hunger works if you want a more fulfilling sex or intimate life.

Most people haven't been taught to fully grasp their holistic sexual experience. So, we'll cover the basics: the roles of your brain and nervous system in sex, the anatomy and science of enhancing pleasure, and how your life experiences affect and are affected by your sex life.

With the foundational structure from Parts 1 and 2, you're building up to use the Arousal Architecture® in Part 3 to help you reach your arousal potential. I'm thrilled to continue this journey with you!

5

Your Brain

Pathways for Better Arousal and Sex

This chapter will help you understand select brain processes to harness their power for overall wellness, stress reduction, and sexual arousal. You'll learn more about the nervous system and the mind-body connection to find ways to make your brain work for you instead of against you. It truly is the key to unlocking healthy sexual exploration and adventure with compassion.

Although these concepts seem relatively straightforward, fully experiencing the benefits can be a complex process and hard to integrate into everyday life. This is challenging for most people because we aren't taught how to do it in ways that resonate with us or that we can quickly implement in our day-to-day lives, even though we should regularly keep nervous system regulation at the forefront of our minds.

The mind-body connection and nervous system regulation are significant parts of the solution for sexual challenges, yet they are commonly overlooked (even by medical doctors). Many healthcare providers forget or don't have time to explain in detail why and how to regulate the nervous system, aside from telling patients to try meditating, get more exercise, or reduce stress.

This is why creating a skill set of Nervous System Awareness and Regulation Techniques is the underlying principle that every single one of my clients has learned in our work together. Without incorporating the nervous system into their treatment, patient efforts to resolve sexual challenges often take longer, or they end up feeling like something is inherently wrong with them.

In this chapter, you'll gain science-based insights to reclaim control over your body and sexual experience. Your brain, your most powerful sex organ, influences arousal, pleasure, and overall wellness more than mere genital stimulation—a revelation for many. We'll delve into how a healthy nervous system fosters sexual arousal and address strategies for managing sexual anxiety and pain, vital steps toward embracing your empowered sexual self. For now, we'll explore how a healthy nervous system creates healthy sexual arousal, as well as what to do when you're feeling sexually anxious or experiencing pain. It will be a crucial step to reclaiming sex and satisfaction while stepping more fully into your empowered sexual self.

Additionally, we'll explore trauma responses in a new light, offering pathways to enhance sexual resiliency, even if trauma isn't part of your story. These insights will complement the lessons you've already learned.

While the nervous system's complexities are vast, this book provides the critical nuggets you need to rewrite your sexual narrative without feeling like you're working on a neurobiology degree.

Your Mind-Body Connection for Sexual Satisfaction

The "mind-body connection" has been studied for centuries and refers to the complex connection between what occurs in our mind and body and how it's related to our physical and mental health. All of it is interconnected. The stronger and more regulated the mind-body connection one has, the easier it is to improve and influence physical and mental well-being. At the same time, healthy physical and mental states enhance the functioning of the mind-body connection, making it easier to build overall wellness and reduce stress.[1]

The World Health Organization defines "stress" in a way that can help us understand two main components:

- A state of worry or tension.
- A typical human response that facilitates us to address challenges and threats in our lives.[2]

Having stress isn't inherently a problem. It's how we deal with stress that causes physical and mental difficulties or even illnesses.

Sexual challenges are frequently caused by and create stress. If left unresolved, they can be hard to overcome. When you're constantly stressed, whether that's about sex or life in general, your nervous system is not likely to create the kind of response your body needs to access arousal or experience pleasure. And when sex isn't occurring the way that makes you feel good, it can increase a stress response.

You must interrupt the process; and you'll learn how through an embodied self-awareness process.

Pop quiz! Thinking about what you've already learned about "embodiment" and "self-awareness," take a moment to reflect on what "embodied self-awareness" means to you. Doing this on your own before continuing to read my explanation will help you deepen your learning by creating even more pathways for the content. Even if you don't think you know, pause and think about what it could mean anyway.

Ready for my opinion? In the context of what we're discussing, "embodied self-awareness" is being present and (mostly) regulated when reflecting on your mental, emotional, and physical states. It also identifies whether you think and behave in ways aligned with your internal standards (values and desires). How close are we in our definitions? Hopefully, they were pretty close. If not, it's okay; we're going to go over a little refresher here anyway.

Being *embodied* is a powerful state where you're able to check in with yourself, listen to your needs and internal experiences, and adjust accordingly (such as through regulating). It's like having a personal compass that guides you. A simple example of being embodied is when you notice you're thirsty and reach for some water to drink, paying attention to how you move your body and the sensations you notice as you pick up the glass, all without creating a story or placing judgment on yourself (such as "Ugh, I keep forgetting to drink water today").

Self-awareness is a superpower that allows you to notice and reflect on how well your thoughts, feelings, and behaviors align with your belief systems and values (internal standards). It's also about being aware of your impact on others.

Continuing with the drinking water example, as you realize you're thirsty, you might notice a desire to reach for your iced latte next to your water. However, you know that you haven't had much water today, which usually results in a headache later in the day. Plus, you know the importance of staying well hydrated. So, you intentionally reach for the water, noticing the sensations as you take a step toward self-love and a healthier body. As a reward, you take a sip of the iced latte, noticing the sensations of yummy joy that the tasty beverage brings you.

As a bonus, I threw that last sentence in there to continue to weave in the concepts you've been learning in multiple ways. What tool do you think I was using there? If you guessed "Noticing Pleasant," you'd be right!

When experiencing embodied self-awareness around sex, you aim to be in alignment with what you want and what's important to you, which is why we first started with unlearning outdated belief systems about sex, intimacy, and relationships.

Another benefit of creating a healthy mind-body connection is understanding when and how to use tools to regulate. Focusing on and increasing your awareness around when you're feeling stressed, anxious, or in pain can feel counter-intuitive. If you're like most of my clients when they start working with me, you probably try to actively avoid those unpleasant feelings, hoping they'll go away or resolve on their own. While that *might* happen sometimes, if you've been dealing with it for a while, it needs to be addressed eventually.

Lucky for you, you're learning the tools to navigate awareness with empowerment instead of avoidance. When confronted with a stressful sexual situation, catch it, have compassion for yourself and your feelings, and then redirect your focus to neutral or pleasant sensations or thoughts. Your aim in using the mind-body connection is to create more self-awareness and allow yourself the space to explore the emotions that arise with non-judgmental compassion.

When you get the hang of embodied self-awareness and your mind-body connection as it relates to sex, you gain more control over your access to sexual arousal and stress caused by sexual experiences. One of the key ingredients is listening to your body's subtle messages (a.k.a. sensations as your body's cues).

The Nervous System for Sexual Wellness and Pleasure

Before learning how you can reduce the impact of sexual and overall stress, it's helpful to learn the structures and functions within your mind-body connection that help you do that.

The nervous system (your brain, spinal cord, and nerves) controls and regulates practically everything we do, from breathing to digesting food to sexual function.

The nervous system has two branches: the *sympathetic nervous system* (also known as the flight-or-fight system) and the *parasympathetic nervous system* (also known as the rest-and-digest system).

We briefly explored how these two systems work together to keep you safe, help you respond to perceived threats, and modify outdated belief systems.

Now, we'll delve deeper into this process regarding sexual functioning so you can really grasp why this is important.

The sympathetic nervous system activates in various ways to help us throughout the day. While you might mostly be familiar with this system as the flight-or-fight response, it's not always activated when there's danger or a threat. For instance, it's also activated when we inhale.

The parasympathetic nervous system helps us with the functions to restore, relax, and recover (including exhaling). Both systems are usually activated simultaneously, one often operating more than the other depending on your body's need at that particular moment. A regulated and healthy nervous system aims to create a harmonious flow between both systems. It can look a little like Figure 5.1.

When someone experiences chronic stress, anxiety, or pain, their sympathetic nervous system (activation) tends to be more active than the parasympathetic nervous system (release). This state, known as the "High Zone," can exacerbate unpleasant experiences and potentially lead to chronic illnesses, particularly when stress hormones like cortisol reach toxic levels. In the context of sexual health and intimacy, an imbalance favoring the flight-or-fight response can

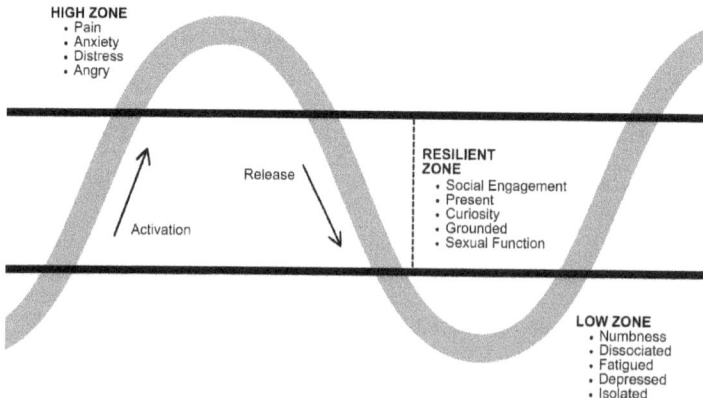

FIGURE 5.1 *Resilient Zone for nervous system activation and release. Adapted from Miller-Karas, Building Resilience.*

result in muscle tension, restricted blood flow, irritability, and other issues that we'll explore shortly.

Bottom line: A healthy and balanced nervous system is the path to increasing sexual arousal, pleasure, and connection.

Have I sold you on the importance of a regulated nervous system? I hope so! If not, I'm sure I'll get there with you shortly.

Wired for Survival, Not Arousal

When you experience something that requires your body to activate the sympathetic nervous system (flight-or-fight response), brain activity, blood flow, and neurochemicals are released to help certain systems in your body turn on or turn off in order to respond to the need. Also, your brain's activity is focused more on surviving or seeking safety, so it's not using its valuable resources for more "evolved" brain activities such as language, logic, or emotionally connecting with another human.

Think about it like this. Imagine you're walking through a jungle, and you come across a tiger. Your system probably has a "short cut" in your brain that has already linked that a tiger in the wild is "dangerous" so it will activate the flight-or-fight response triggering blood flow to your major muscle groups (such as your legs, arms, and core), so you are prepared to run or fight if needed. Your system will also allocate energy and resources from systems that are not necessary for survival in that moment, such as digestion, having a rational or connected conversation with the person next to you, or sexual arousal.

When this happens in your nervous system, you may feel muscle tension, an increased heart rate, shallow breathing, or mental fog. These sensations are caused by the release of cortisol and adrenaline in your body, which trigger a heightened sympathetic nervous system response. Recognizing these cues can help you identify when you are feeling stressed and take steps to manage it.

Let's go back to the jungle example. You've been able to run away from that part of the jungle and you finally feel safe. The parasympathetic nervous system becomes more active again and you notice different sensations (cues) occurring as your blood flow, chemical activity, and brain activity release the need for trying to keep you safe and move into putting your body's resources back into recovering and digesting. That might feel like waves of different temperatures, tingles as your muscles release, or the ability to take bigger or deeper breaths.

Now, the next time you go into that part of the jungle, your nervous system remembers the scary experience, and even though there's a 1 in 10,000 chance the tiger will be there again, you can't help but notice that your body is responding to the potential threat as you experience those cues (sensations) popping up again. Your brain does this to keep you safe and create a quicker path to survival in case it's that unlucky chance again that you come face to face with the mighty beast. While your brain is scanning for a likely threat, it's much harder for you to walk through that jungle and easily notice the beauty of it, have a light-hearted conversation with your friend as you walk, or be as present as you were before your tiger encounter.

Remember this formula?

Event + Unpleasant Consequence = Threat = Aversion/Avoidance

Similarly, when sex and dating have been regularly fraught with heavy guilt, shame, and disappointment, our brains build neuropathways that tell us that sex and anything that "looks like" sex (e.g., kissing, sensual touching, etc.) is a perceived threat. The Sexual Aversion Cycle, which we'll explore in a moment, is built and fortified by these neuropathways, especially if the outcome of attempting anything sexual results in unpleasant experiences. Your brain and body have created a shortcut in response to sex and arousal that triggers an "alarm" when it detects what your brain perceives as a threat. Even if you know you love your partner and want to have a close and intimate physical connection with them, your brain has had enough experiences in the past that have told it something sexual or intimate has caused emotional or physical problems in the past. Your brain is only trying to protect you and thinks it's keeping you safe from impending emotionally or physically painful feelings. It thinks it's an act of self-preservation to turn off your sexual response system.

I'll bet my bottom dollar that what you've been told about a "sex drive" is wrong. A biological "drive" is something your body is inherently born to seek out and respond to automatically, the way we do for food and water. It's what our bodies need to stay alive. Instead, sexual desire and arousal are more like reward systems, and if your brain has received the message repeatedly that sex is likely going to be stressful, painful, or disappointing, you can bet your sweet tushie your brain is going to want to save you from continuously experiencing a "threatening" situation. It might even shut down the arousal system and keep you from being motivated for sex, which will make it even more challenging to feel "spontaneous arousal" and much less likely for pleasurable possibilities with sex. You might not even realize that your nervous system is doing this, which is why it's imperative to increase your mind-body connection and self-awareness so that you can detect when your system is starting to work against you by saving you from a perceived threat.

Since our brains are hardwired to keep us safe over being intimate or increasing sexual arousal, it will choose the former. It's an incredibly frustrating (if not downright devastating) process. However, knowing that this is an example of a learned response, it means that you can also unlearn your brain's knee-jerk reaction to sexual aversion and arousal shutdown.

Just like with rewriting your sexual narrative by changing the way you relate to outdated belief systems, the goal here is to create new brain pathways that help you feel more in control by noticing when your flight-or-fight response is becoming activated and pairing those moments with mindfulness or somatic techniques that regulate your nervous system.

The Sexual Aversion Cycle

Remember learned responses? That's the starting point leading into a Sexual Aversion Cycle, which you can see illustrated in Figure 5.2. When you have experienced any consistent physical or emotional suffering around sex, it's going to make sex seem very unappealing. So naturally, when the topic or possibility of sex comes up, you might find yourself wanting to withdraw from sexual activities, dating, or from your partner.

And so, the cycle begins.

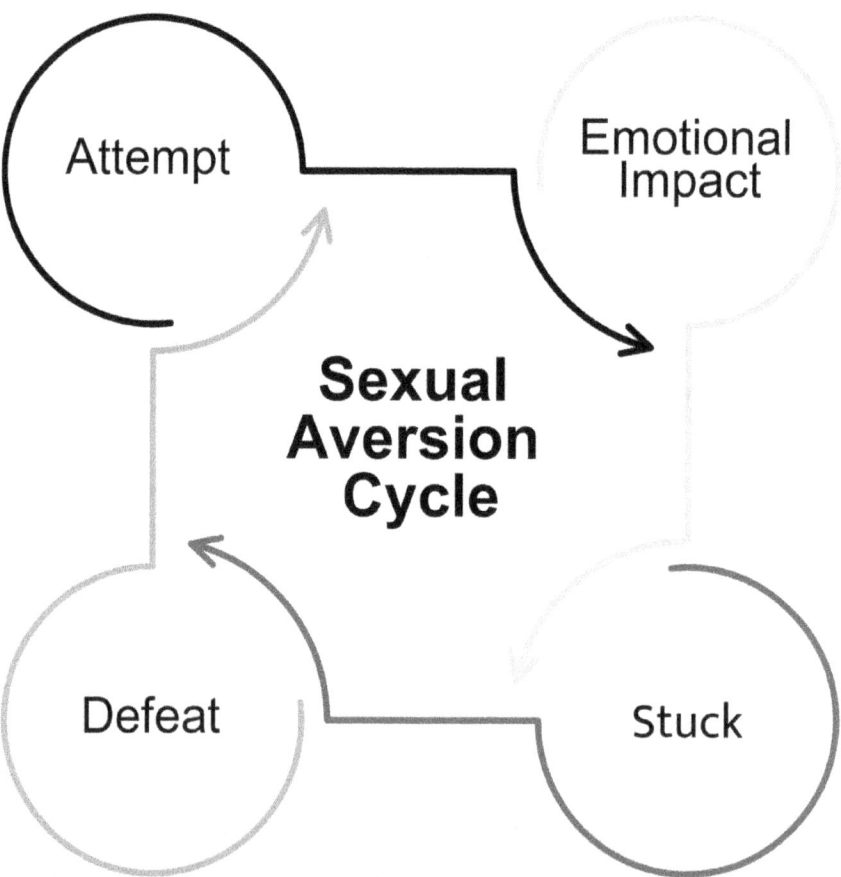

FIGURE 5.2 *The Sexual Aversion Cycle.*

Your brain starts a process that informs your body and mind (subconsciously) to withdraw from sex. It will even go a step further and make things like completing everything on your task list or doing your taxes more appealing than sex. This way, you're protected from confronting the torture of facing a failed sexual experience yet again.

Here's what it might look like to experience this cycle:

- *Attempt*: You might say: "It's been ## days (weeks) & I should probably try." But then it doesn't work because sexual anxiety or pain negatively impacts the attempt.

- *Emotional Impact*: You may experience disappointment, sadness, guilt, or hopelessness. You may feel slightly motivated to change things, which may delay your progress to the next stage.

- *Stuck*: You find yourself in the same conversations with your partner, yourself, or a professional about how to fix it. Nothing changes; you don't arrive at any solutions or don't feel like you can take any other action.

- *Defeat*: You avoid or ignore it until you can't anymore, and you start to feel the pressure or self-criticism moving you back into the cycle again.

I call it an aversive reaction because the way many folks feel about it is beyond simple avoidance. It's a more potent emotional cycle since they have attached emotions like guilt or shame to their experience, especially if the nervous system is highly activated or dysregulated.

Using this tangible model to represent what's happening for you can help you determine the stage you're in and identify interventions to use.

Here are some interventions you could try using to stop the cycle based on the skills you've learned in this book:

1. *Attempt*: Mindset interventions along with nervous system regulation tools to help you with pivoting or growing beyond your comfort zone with embodied perseverance.

2. *Emotional Impact*: Mindfulness, somatic practices, and being a scientist to regulate emotions and increase compassion.

3. *Stuck*: Any of the interventions can help, along with the effective communication skills you'll learn about in Part 4.

4. *Defeat*: Pivoting and Redirecting to Neutral or Pleasant to identify different ways to try something different or create alternative possibilities.

What Happens to Your Sexual System When Stressed or Anxious

Being in a dysregulated or chronically stressed state that activates the flight-or-fight response will reduce resources in the body that are important to sexual arousal, pleasure, and orgasm. Mainly, we're talking about muscle contraction, blood flow, lubrication, and the ability to be emotionally and physically present.

Healthy blood flow can create pleasant tingly sensations in the genitals, lubrication, and erection. When in a regulated state, your muscles are properly contracting and releasing which moves blood flow in and out of your pelvic area. Additionally, if you have proper contraction and release, you'll more easily obtain lubrication or erection. On top of that, muscle contraction and release is part of the process that creates an orgasm: your muscles contract and release repeatedly, while blood flow moves around, and eventually your body releases all the muscle tension that's built up in your pelvic area (and sometimes your whole body), leading to a heightened wave of pleasure and relaxation.

If you're in a chronically stressed state, you might not be able to have proper muscle contraction or release, lubrication and erection tend to be reduced, and orgasm could feel more challenging or less satisfying. Furthermore, being in a dysregulated state reduces the ability to be present with whatever you're doing and limits connection with others. So, if your sympathetic nervous system is activated and you're attempting to engage with a partner sexually, you won't be able to connect emotionally as well (or at all). Even if you're having casual sex and you don't want deep emotional connection with your partner (which is completely normal and can be a very healthy way to have sex), you still might not be able to tune into your pleasure needs or notice what's happening for your partner. Being able to access your internal experience and stay connected to who you're having sex with improves the experience overall.

Physically and Emotionally Painful Sex Creates a Threat Response

Trauma can be a heavy topic. However, it's essential to address in this book not only because of its significance on its own but also because when I learned about somatically based trauma reprocessing as a psychotherapy treatment modality, I realized that sexual challenges are similar to a threat or trauma response in the body as someone who experiences a trauma trigger—they both go into flight-or-fight modes (sometimes even freeze). They also engage in avoidance patterns along with a variety of other similar responses.

Not only did these revelations change the work I was doing with clients who acknowledged trauma as a part of their past, but also because a lot of people don't realize their experiences could qualify as trauma. For instance, something seemingly unrelated to sex (like "perfectionism") can create a trauma response in the body that impacts sexual arousal indirectly, as we have discussed, or directly because someone who's aiming to be perfect might have fears of "letting go," making it harder for them to achieve an orgasm or erection when they want.

We're used to conceptualizing traumas that are referred to as "Big T" Traumas, such as the following:

- Abuse (verbal, physical, emotional, or sexual)
- Neglect as a child
- Alcoholism or substance addiction (either someone's own or that of someone in the household)
- Being in a deadly car accident, but being the only survivor or one of the survivors
- Living in poverty
- Being in a combat zone
- Experiencing a natural disaster

"Little t" traumas are like silent storms that can leave a lasting impact. They are situations where someone has experienced significant distress, yet there was no apparent violence or disaster. These traumas can be very sneaky, often going unnoticed or unacknowledged.

Over the years, I've heard clients consider the following as their "little t" traumas (some of them can also be Big T Traumas):

- Falls or accidents
- Dental procedures
- Losing something important (like a passport)
- Minor car accidents

Regardless of how these experiences might be categorized, any of them can be experienced as a significant trauma. Below are some traumas my clients have shared that have landed in their bodies as Big T Traumas—do any resonate with you?

- Perfectionism
- Purity culture

- Negative sex messages
- A breakup
- Intimate or romantic betrayal (such as being cheated on or lied to)

The point of the distinction in these categories is to broaden our understanding of what trauma is since most of us typically think of it in terms of significant Big T events (such as horrible abuse). In my trauma therapy certification program with the Trauma Resource Institute, I first heard them describe trauma as something that's "too little, or too much, for too long."[3] Sexual challenges can certainly feel like something that causes feelings or beliefs that are too much or not enough for too long, especially when it comes to emotions like shame, guilt, or significant disappointment.

Even if having "trauma" doesn't resonate with you, it can be helpful to conceptualize sexual challenges like "trauma responses" (or at least threat responses). After all, if you've been having sexual difficulties for a while, your system has probably begun to view "sex" as a "threat," as mentioned in the previous sections. Your nervous system might be responding similarly as it would when experiencing a trauma trigger or threat.

Although some adverse experiences need proper trauma resolution and treatment, other interventions using the body and its sensations to resolve psychological challenges are not limited to psychotherapy. The main principle of resolving trauma is to help the nervous system feel safe and in control. This creates a sense of safety through amplifying cues (sensations) or experiences reinforcing safety and empowerment.

Lucky for you, you're building these skills and implementing these interventions already. You will continue to do this as you read, whether your system is having a trauma response or not. The process you've been practicing in this book gives you a system and tangible techniques that provide structure, and structure offers a sense of safety. Having these to rely on when you experience everything from pre-date jitters to sexual anxiety or pain to full-blown trauma triggers helps create a container for those big emotions. It can give you a sense of control, knowing you have tools to implement and how to use them best. This overarching skill set is building resilience, which you've already been doing a lot of, and soon you'll learn how to create and amplify sexual resiliency.

What If You've Had Trauma?

Sometimes, folks who have had difficulties with sexual experiences and relationships know or realize that Big T Trauma is one piece of their sexual puzzle. A person might have had sexual, physical, emotional, or even covert trauma causing a lot of difficulties in sex. At the core of a healthy sexual experience, a person needs to feel generally safe, in control, and respected. Having a past with unresolved trauma means that a person's nervous system is constantly seeking safety, such as being in a fight/flight mode or shutting down. It's difficult accessing sexual arousal when someone is in survival mode.

Folks who have dealt with any trauma, and particularly Big T Trauma, will likely struggle to respond with a partner, sexually and emotionally. Somatically focused trauma treatment and structured sexual context that provides safety cues are imperative to rewrite sexual narratives when dealing with Big T Trauma.[4]

Maybe some of the previous resonated with you. Or, as you move through this book, perhaps some realization comes to you, and you discover that you've also experienced some form of significant trauma. If this happens to you, first of all, I empathize. As someone who's experienced trauma, I know how difficult it can be to navigate through daily life sometimes, let alone deal with the impact it has on your sex life.

Second, rely on the skills in this book we've already explored or get the support of a qualified, certified trauma therapist who primarily uses somatic modalities. If you need further resources, I've included several at the back of the book.

Use Your Body's Resources to Regulate Your Nervous System for Sex

Let's explore how to identify when and how to regulate your nervous system. Spoiler alert—you already know a lot of this! Now, you'll apply it to sex, arousal, and pleasure.

Before we move forward, let's take a moment to reinforce some key points:

- Mindfulness creates present-moment awareness and regulates your nervous system with the mind-body connection.

- Somatic sensations are internal body-based responses from emotions or experiences happening to or around you.

- Learned responses are repeated experiences that create a seemingly automatic response or a belief system. These responses can often be unlearned, leading to new brain pathways and possibilities.

When you become more aware of your mind and body's state regarding sex, you'll notice cues or sensations associated with stress or anxiety and those that indicate you're feeling more regulated. These sensations often occur just below our consciousness, so bringing them to the surface takes practice. Sensations usually happen before we even identify an emotion, so recognizing these cues can help you use regulation techniques before feeling hijacked by them.

Figure 5.3 illustrates a concept from the Trauma Resource Institute that shows how someone with a *narrow* Resilient Zone gets "bumped out" during stressful stimuli while someone with a *broader* Resilient Zone remains regulated (even if moderately activated). By noticing your body's cues of dysregulation, you can use nervous system regulation techniques to stay within and widen your Resilient Zone over time.

For example, imagine feeling (self-inflicted) pressured to have sex whenever your partner suggests it, leading to unpleasant experiences. Over time,

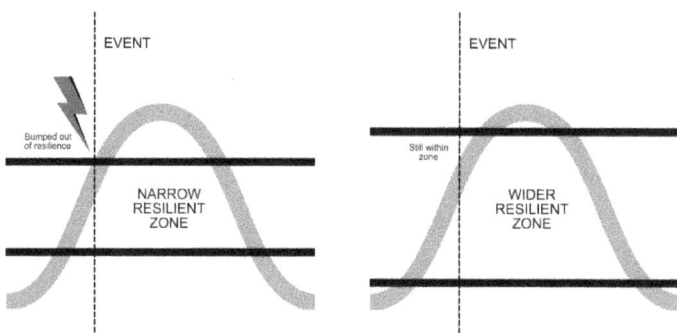

FIGURE 5.3 *Narrow and wide Resilient Zone comparisons of the same event or stimulus. Adapted from Miller-Karas,* Building Resilience.

whenever your partner comes in for a longer-than-usual kiss indicating they want to go to sexy town, your body braces for the inevitable Sexual Aversion Cycle. This has caused you to withdraw from overtly intimate moments and maybe even to ignore other ways your partner expresses desire.

With self-awareness and the right tools, you can interrupt this cycle. By recognizing your nervous system's response early, you can activate regulation techniques before the cycle starts.

Below is a step-by-step process to regain control over your body and sex life. It may seem straightforward, but practically implementing it can be challenging, so be kind to yourself and make space for imperfect practice.

1. Engage in sexual conversations, experiences, or arousal techniques.
2. Create awareness around your nervous system's cues.
3. Utilize nervous system regulation techniques.
4. Redirect to neutral or pleasant sensations.

We've been layering lessons, concepts, and skills to apply them in multiple situations—first in non-sexual ways, then regarding outdated beliefs about sexuality, and finally in sexual experiences.

When encountering unpleasant emotions, thoughts, or behaviors in a sexual situation, start with non-judgmental self-awareness. Approach it with curiosity to understand what happened and find ways to improve the experience next time.

Deepening your awareness of your mind-body connection will help you notice when you're becoming dysregulated. Use the tools we've discussed to stay in the Resilient Zone and stop the Sexual Aversion Cycle. By focusing on neutral or pleasant sensations when shifting or stopping the cycle, you reinforce those pathways and increase sexual resiliency. The more you do this, the more you create new brain pathways that tell your brain and body that sex is not a threat.

Building Sexual Resiliency

With the new perspectives I offer in this book and tools and models such as the Arousal Architecture®, you'll build what I described as "sexual resiliency." Resiliency (also referred to as "resilience") is the ability to recover quickly from difficulties or adversities.

One thing my clients find so powerful in our work is how we're able to hone in on their abilities to be resilient in areas outside of sex and intimacy and then apply those skills to sexual situations. It's how I've also been able to shorten my client's treatment time—it's a sexual healing life hack!

You can do this, too, by identifying what you know you already do well and applying those skill sets to sexual and intimate experiences. For instance, if you know that you're able to carry out difficult tasks at work and complete your assignments on time because you have scheduled time in your work calendar to achieve them, then you might think about using that same tactic when it comes to integrating some of the exercises I'll teach you in this book.

Sexual resiliency is a crucial aspect of sexual healing. Most people need to be taught how to handle rejection well. Often, we see a situation as a rejection, but it's not. We need to learn to hear our partner's "not right now" as an invitation to pivot, collaborate, or be inspired to connect in other ways that are a "heck yes!" for everyone involved.

My clients also learn that their "no" to sex or sexual experiences sometimes means they don't have another way to ask for what they truly want, and "no" is the easiest way to protect themselves from guilt, disappointment, or shame. Learning how to tolerate discomfort around sex and intimacy in a regulated way is how you will build sexual resiliency.

Side note: A "no" can always mean "no" without explanation or doubt. *Always* listen to someone when they say "no." Enthusiastic consent is sexy for everyone involved. If you feel like your "no" has ever been pushed, coerced, or completely bulldozed, or you had experiences where you never gave a "yes" and someone did something anyway, it can be complicated to deal with. If you haven't worked through that experience from a somatic lens with a qualified trauma therapist or practitioner, you might benefit from somatically focused trauma treatment.

As you continue to shift your perspectives and belief systems from outdated concepts that have kept you back while rewiring your brain for pleasure using the tools and systems in this book designed to empower you, your sexual resiliency will expand and make it easier and easier to rewrite your sexual narrative.

Creating Alternative Possibilities

Expanding sexual resiliency provides your brain with new empowered ways of thinking about situations and yourself.

With that, you can begin to identify "Alternative Possibilities" more easily. The parts of your brain that are used for higher-level thinking beyond just surviving help facilitate empathy, logic, language, and social connection. When you're in regulated states and have access to these parts of your brain, you can create alternative meanings and compassionate understanding around what's happening instead of the default you're probably used to (self-criticism, self-consciousness, shame, guilt, disappointment, etc.).

Being able to identify new perspectives supports rewriting your sexual narratives to the different possibilities and belief systems that are now available to you when you might not have realized they were even there.

With the exercises in this chapter, you can identify and enhance opportunities for increased sexual resiliency.

Pleasure Gems

- Your mind-body connection is vital to overall wellness, stress reduction, and sexual arousal. It truly is one of the keys to unlocking healthy sexual exploration and adventure with compassion.

- Knowing how your brain and nervous system function and facilitating a healthy mind-body connection will help you rewrite your sexual narrative by building sexual resiliency and creating Alternative Possibilities.

- You also learned that your brain wants to follow the path of least resistance to perceived safety. This is similar to the way your brain handles a threat or trauma response, so we're using that perspective to make it easier to access arousal and sexual pleasure on a cellular level.

Exercises

Quick Win!

Build Resiliency Awareness

Take a moment to notice (or even start to write a list of) the sensations in your body that you experience when you're feeling resilient.

Refer to the Sensations List if you need help with possible sensations you might feel. It's different for everyone, but when I'm in a state of resiliency, I notice an expansion in my chest and back; a calm, open mind; a central column in my core that inspires me to stand tall; a smile on my lips; and a playful and curious energy that's best described as tingles moving pleasantly through my body.

If you need practice experiencing resiliency or you don't even know what it feels like for you, recall a moment when you overcame something challenging. It doesn't have to deal with sex; it can be anything you have accomplished. Or reflect on a time when you were proud of how you handled a situation or a conversation. As you think about it, notice the sensations that occur.

Resiliency sensations are often similar to what you might feel when you're present with pleasant sensations. Spend thirty seconds or more feeling those sensations within your body. Refer to the somatic practices in Part 1 that helped you connect more with your pleasant sensations. These practices can lay the foundation for connecting to resiliency more easily.

Going Deeper

Actively Create Alternative Possibilities

With this exercise, you will expand on the exercises from Part 1. Identify automatic thoughts or Limiting Beliefs that you have about your body, sexual arousal, or pleasure. Writing them down can help you keep track of them and create objectivity.

Use this prompt: "An outdated belief or unpleasant thought I have about sex, intimacy, or pleasure is . . ."

If writing multiple beliefs or automatic thoughts, give yourself space between each one for a future step.

Notice what's happening in your body as you do this part of the exercise. If you find that you're feeling slightly or fully dysregulated, utilize your mindfulness or somatic tools! Move forward once you feel mostly neutral or regulated in your mind and body. Since you're rewiring these patterns in your brain, the pathways will be more challenging to pave if you're in a dysregulated or disembodied state.

Once you acknowledge that you feel primarily neutral or pleasant, write an Alternative Possibility under each automatic thought or belief you wrote.

Use this prompt to help: "One day, I can imagine myself thinking, feeling, or believing this . . . [write the more empowered, present, excited, pleasurable version of the outdated belief or unpleasant thought]."

When you identify an Alternative Possibility, notice sensations or what happens in your body. Pay closer attention to the neutral or pleasant sensations or places in your body that believe this possibility could exist for you.

6

Your Body

Sexual Anatomy and Pleasure Science

Orange Is the New Black is an iconic show for many reasons. One scene in particular has always stuck out in my memory. In season 2, episode 4, some of the cisgender women in the prison realized they were clueless about their genitalia. I loved that Sophia (who is a transwoman in the show and real life, played by Laverne Cox) provided the much-needed sexual health education to the other inmates about how many holes a vulva has, their biological terms, and what each one is for. In case you're also unclear about these parts and functions, that's what this chapter is for!

I've heard from many clients and others that they aren't confident about their (or their partner's) genitalia either. Society, fear- or shame-based sex education, and oppressive mainstream porn have not taught us well. We've also been told there's a standard of beauty for genitals, making most of us doubt how well our bodies measure up. There's a lot of pressure about having a "beautiful" or "sexy" body, forgetting that beauty is in the eye of the beholder.

Knowing the names and functions of your parts and the parts of people you're sexual with increases arousal potential, sexual confidence, and satisfaction. Pleasure is much more possible when you know what parts of your body like to be touched, when, and how. Beyond that, it's also highly satisfying to communicate this to partners, and it opens doors to more profound sexual satisfaction for everyone involved.

In this chapter, I'll teach the basics of genital anatomy and what happens to our bodies when sexually aroused. This book wouldn't be complete without mentioning some parts of our bodies that can amplify pleasure. You'll also gain insight into the science of pleasure and powerful models to maximize transformation.

Becoming Friends with Your Body

The first and most important benefit of knowing about the anatomy of your body is that you will understand what feels best for your body and when. Knowing what your body enjoys and what it needs to feel pleasure, arousal, and orgasm is a healthy gift of self-love.

Self-Pleasuring Practices

One of the best ways to get to know yourself is through masturbation. There are a lot of belief systems that say self-pleasure or masturbation is dirty, shameful, and even sinful. Some of those systems are steeped in oppression, and some of those systems are based on religious and cultural expectations. Most American school systems teach sex-negative education. Many young folks walk away with discomfort, disgust, or shame attached to typical human responses such as sexual arousal, masturbation, and sexual preference.

Unfortunately, masturbation is still a controversial topic and figuring out how you feel about self-pleasuring and why you feel that way can be a crucial part of your sexually empowering journey.

For instance, suppose you find yourself in a conflict, knowing that masturbation can be a healthy expression of self-love, but your culture or religion tells you differently. In that case, you could explore how to maintain the core values and lifestyle that are essential aspects of traditional beliefs while finding alignment with your values that also embrace typical human development, self-expression with what you do with your own body, and scientific findings that support masturbation as a healthy sexual practice.[1] If you find yourself in that place, that's where the exercises in the first part of the book can come in handy, or working with a secular, evidence-based sex therapist to support you as you navigate the process with someone who won't insert their beliefs or biases into your therapeutic work.

In full transparency, I am personally biased toward science and research. Masturbation is objectively healthy. However, many readers have strong beliefs and discomfort with it. I'll provide accessible information to support your sexually empowered journey, no matter your beliefs. The focus is on building pathways to pleasure, even beyond the genitals.

Research shows that self-pleasure can regulate the nervous system and reduce anxiety and stress.[2] It's like a self-massage on pleasurable steroids. However, reasons for masturbation can vary and might feel exciting or painful, like if it's compulsive or a substitute for a partner. This book aims to help you feel good in both body and mind about engaging in pleasure-based self-love.

Self-pleasuring doesn't have to involve only the genitals. Including other body parts can be a calming technique, helping you understand what kind of touch you like. If you don't know what you enjoy, it's challenging for a partner to help you find or experience pleasure. Many people expect their partners to know what they like instinctively, which creates pressure for everyone. Understanding your preferences and communicating them fosters sexual empowerment.

For example, one client discovered she enjoyed nipple stimulation only when she was already aroused. After discussing this with her partner, they developed a plan to signal her readiness. This simple conversation improved their sexual experience.

Consent is crucial before touching or discussing someone's body. Explicit permission ensures everyone is on board, increasing pleasure and connection. Asking your partner about their likes and dislikes is a brave step in building an embodied sexual relationship. Not to mention super sexy. Healthy conversations about sex lead to more satisfying experiences and improved sexual well-being.[3]

Preferences can change based on mood, stress, or cycle phases. For instance, some people dislike light touch when stressed but love it otherwise.

Using consent-based language during sexual play can be highly arousing and connecting. Simple questions like "Does that feel nice?" or "Do you want more or less?" can enhance the experience. If verbal communication feels challenging, consider asking your partner these questions in advance:

- How would I know you like something during sexual play?
- What movements or sounds indicate you don't like something?
- Are there off-limits areas for touching during sexual play?
- What types of touch do you absolutely love?

Communicating during sexual activities helps provide constructive feedback and ensures a supportive, connected experience. Part 4 will guide you through communicating effectively about sex and preferences.

The goal of this chapter is to inspire you to become friends with your body, especially the parts that bring sexual pleasure. Understanding your anatomy and others' helps navigate pleasure centers. Our sex-negative culture often disconnects us from our bodies and genitals. Overcoming these barriers starts with learning about your anatomy and neutrally connecting with your body.

Imagine your genitals are strangers that you would like to get to know; the first thing you might do is offer to have coffee or tea with them. Now, I know you're not going to take your genitals out in a coffee shop; however, think about your genitals much the same way. Approach them with curiosity, non-judgment, and compassion no matter what your history is with your genitals or body overall.

If you feel uncomfortable or disgusted by your genitals, understand that this is common. Use your tools to maintain self-awareness and regulate your nervous system if you feel activated while reading this chapter. After thirty to sixty seconds of engaging in the practice, notice the change, paying particular attention to the places in your body that feel more neutral or pleasant. Then, continue reading or engage in a longer regulating practice.

Engaging in self-aware embodiment while reading about sex rewires your brain's pathways. Creating positive, neutral, or pleasant pathways helps you feel more sexually empowered and excited for possibilities.

Pelvic Floor Muscles

Are you familiar with your pelvic floor? If not, you're not alone! I've been surprised at how many sexual self-help books fail to talk about the pelvic floor muscles, even though that muscle group is responsible for so much of our arousal and pleasure.

As you can see illustrated in Figure 6.1, your pelvic floor is like a hammock of muscles in your pelvic area. They span the area from hip bone to hip bone and tailbone to pubic bone. The pelvic floor muscles hold up all your lower abdomen organs for healthy digestive, reproductive, and sexual functioning.

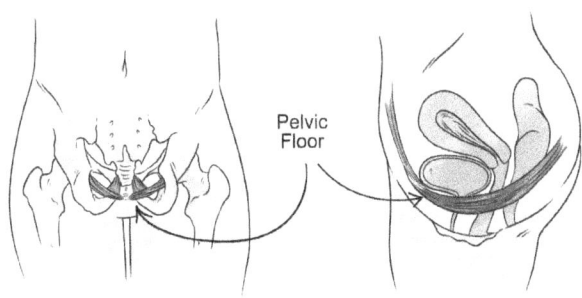

FIGURE 6.1 *Pelvic floor front (left) and side (right) views.*

Your pelvic floor muscles contribute to sexual wellness. For instance, they contract and release to move blood to your genitals and help facilitate lubrication and genital engorgement (such as erections or increased clitoral sensitivity).

The pelvic floor coordinates with the core muscles and other body parts for healthy sexual functioning. When there's a discoordination between the pelvic floor and core muscles, it can result in pelvic floor dysfunction.

If the muscles are too tight, they can cause muscle pain or myalgia and limit blood flow in the hips and pelvic area. A tight pelvic floor can also impact other body parts, causing deferred pain or other structural problems. You can even get knots in your pelvic floor that a pelvic floor physical therapist could address, just like if you had a knot in your back and sought care from a massage therapist.

Contrary to popular belief, many people think everyone should be doing Kegels, but that's not always the case and can create more problems than they help. Always get a professional's opinion before doing Kegels or using things like yoni or jade eggs.

However, some people need strengthening in their pelvic floor muscles; otherwise, different muscle groups like your back or hips could overcompensate, causing other structural issues or pain in your body.

Pelvic floor dysfunction can cause sexual pain, incontinence, constipation, or irritative bladder symptoms, among other (sometimes surprising) medical challenges. If the pelvic floor is not adequately functioning, it can also lead to difficulty becoming aroused and experiencing orgasm.[4]

To treat pelvic floor dysfunction, you would see a pelvic floor physical therapist. They are Doctors of Physical Therapy who obtain specialized training and experience in treating the pelvic floor. Most people are about as familiar with pelvic floor physical therapists as they are with sex therapists in that most people don't realize they exist, let alone know how beneficial a healthcare professional they can be. As a person who has experienced pelvic floor physical therapy myself and has many colleagues who collaborate on client cases with me, I can attest to the wonderful and much-needed support they can provide for sexual well-being.

Case Study: Jessica (she/her)

Jessica struggled with orgasm, and although she worked with a physical therapist, she was still having difficulty. This wasn't because physical therapy wasn't effective; she needed it because her pelvic floor and core muscles were discoordinated, possibly contributing to a structural issue that could have been a factor in her ability to orgasm. However, Jessica's anxiety and fear were also creating struggles in reaching orgasm. Since our brains are incredibly powerful, it's possible that her fear and anxiety around sex and orgasm occurred very early on in her life. Her body received the message that sexual pleasure and orgasms were "scary" or a threat, so her brain taught her muscles to stop contracting properly. This is what's called a *psychosomatic response*—Jessica's body created an expression of her fear of "letting go" through a physical symptom. While we might never truly know if this was the case for Jessica, it's the reason having a multifaceted treatment team of mental and medical professionals is crucial for overcoming sexual challenges.

Thorough pelvic floor physical therapists help patients by examining the pelvic floor internally (through the vagina or rectum). They also observe how a patient moves and other structural assessments to understand the whole picture of a patient's body. Pelvic floor physical therapists don't only use internal work to address the dysfunction; they can also help patients find stretches and strengthening exercises for the rest of the body to help the pelvic floor obtain the proper coordination a patient's body needs.

If you think you have challenges with pelvic floor dysfunction, seek out a local pelvic floor physical therapist, or you can reach out to me because I have an extensive network of folks that I trust.

The most important thing for you to know is that if you are having sexual challenges, a physical therapist could be a great addition to your treatment team. Insurance companies cover some pelvic floor physical therapists. However, if you find a therapist that's not covered, they are probably worth the investment.

External Genitalia

Most people are familiar with the concept of "male and female" genitals, the most common chromosomal expression and appearance of genitals. People who have been assigned a sex that also matches their gender are called "cisgender" (also cis man or cis woman); you might use the term "man" or "woman" but expanding your understanding for more inclusive language around biological sex (e.g., male, female, intersex) and gender is important. We'll talk about the difference between sex and gender in a moment.

There are many beautiful parts of the genitals—knowing the name of yours and your partner's is vital for sexual pleasure. I have highlighted the parts of the genitals that we're most familiar with and typically interact with when being sexual. However, this is not an exhaustive list and not the same for everyone; I encourage you to explore as much as you want, wherever you want, while figuring out what feels pleasing for you (or your partners).

Genitalia: Your Parts and Parts of Partners (Possibly)

Biological sex has been studied for decades, and there have been significant understandings about what biological sex and gender genuinely are. Since the depth of exploring these concepts and the multi-layered findings in research around biological sex are beyond the scope of this book, I'll discuss the most common genetic expressions and anatomical terms found in external genitalia as they relate to sexual activities and pleasure.

Since most folks are born with most of these parts, the descriptions that follow are meant to be inclusive to all genders, recognizing that there may be some variations for some folks, especially those who identify as intersex, trans (transsexuals), and non-binary. There is so much more to the language we use around biological sex, anatomy, and gender. Regardless of how you identify or which parts you have, I hope that what you read feels validating and supportive. If you think I could do better, please reach out—I always love expanding and understanding better!

On cis women and bodies with vulvas, the external genital area that most people call the "vagina" is actually called the "vulva."

As you can see in Figure 6.2, the *vulva* consists of all the external genitals: *the outer and inner labia, clitoris, urethra,* and *vaginal opening.*

The *vagina* has its own internal structure consisting of the *vaginal canal* and the *vaginal opening.* The vaginal opening is typically where tampons, sex toys, fingers, or penises might be inserted (although some of those items might also be inserted into other genital holes). The vaginal canal extends into the body, and when aroused, the canal elongates, and the internal organs (*cervix* and *uterus*) tuck up into the body to accommodate whatever's being inserted. This

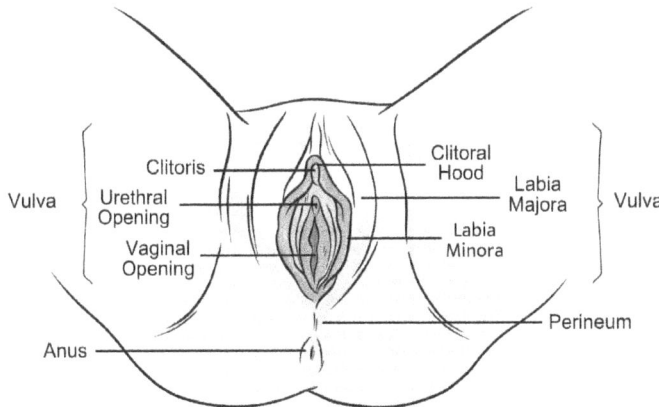

FIGURE 6.2 *Vulva and external genitals splayed apart with labels for potential pleasure centers.*

process is why some people experience pain when not sufficiently aroused before inserting something inside of the vagina; they might be hitting the tip of the cervix or a tender muscle if their body hasn't had time to expand and relax before insertion. Warming up is crucial!

When most people talk about the "lips," they are referring to the *outer labia* (*labia majora*) and *inner labia* (*labia minora*), which are the layers of vulvar skin that make up the two layers of protective tissue around the clitoris, urethra, and vaginal opening. Some people have long labia, others have short, and some have different lengths on each side. There is a wide range of labia colors, even within the same vulva. No scientific data says that one formation is better, even though most mainstream porn makes us think that it's normal for labia to be short or petite and light-skinned. This is simply not accurate and another way society puts pressure on us and reinforces harmful belief systems like misogyny and racism.

If you or your partner has a vulva, it is beautiful, no matter how it looks. Check out a fantastic website called "All Vulvas Are Beautiful" (made popular by *Sex Education* on Netflix), where you can see illustrations of various vulvas and their differences in shape, size, and color to help bust the shame many folks attach to their or others' vulvas.[5]

The *clitoris* (or "clit") is considered the hub of pleasure centers in most bodies with vulvas. Although most people think the clit is only the tiny structure just above the urethra, it's actually much more extensive and significant to pleasure (you'll read more about this shortly). The part that most people are used to seeing and calling the clit is the "clitoral head," and is a similar structure to the penis head. Some folks have prominent clits that can always be seen, whereas others might be tucked back under the clitoral hood, and some might just peek out. The *clitoral hood* is a collection of skin that covers the clitoris; however, how much it covers differs from person to person.

A few parts have the same name but are in different places on the body when comparing bodies with vulvas and bodies with penises.

The *urethra* is the part of the vulva and penis that urine comes out of. In a penis, this is also the opening that ejaculate is released from. For some people, stimulation of the urethral opening and urethral tube can be very pleasurable—but make sure to ask because others can be overly sensitive and not enjoy intentional and direct stimulation there.

The *perineum* is the area between the anus and scrotum or vulva. Both light and firm pressure can enhance pleasure for many people. And the *anus* is the furthest opening front to back in the genitals.

The *penis* consists of the *head* (or *glans*), *foreskin*, *urethra*, and *shaft*, as you see in Figure 6.3. The head typically has more sensitive nerve endings than any other part of the genitals of cis men or bodies with penises.

Penis size can create concerns about self-esteem, sexual play capabilities, and body image. Research from surveys of over 55,000 men found that the average penis size when flaccid is 3.43 inches (8.7 cm), and when erect, 5.48 inches (13.9 cm).[6] Anxiety around penis size is a relatively modern pressure, considering that research found that women did not consider penis size to be the primary determinant of sexual satisfaction.[7] This aligns with my professional experience—I've been helping people with sexual challenges

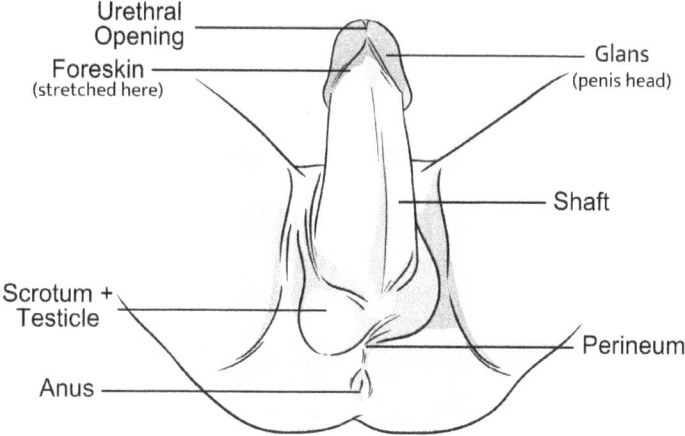

FIGURE 6.3 *Penis and external genitals with legs splayed apart with labels for potential pleasure centers*

since 2006, and most (like 99.99 percent) of folks who have sex with people with penises are more focused on other aspects of sexual play than the size of the penis. As the saying goes, "It's not the size of the ship that matters; it's the motion of the ocean." Pressure and anxiety around penis size is yet another harmful belief system that needs uprooting!

The *foreskin* is the sleeve of skin that extends from the shaft of the penis and surrounds the head. In uncircumcised folks, the foreskin covers the head of the penis while flaccid, and when the penis becomes erect, the foreskin retracts, and the head is exposed. This tissue is similar to the tissue of a clitoral hood on vulvas.

There are a lot of misconceptions about circumcised and uncircumcised penises, and this can bring up self-conscious feelings and even shame for penis owners. Contrary to what most people think, neither is more objectively healthy or hygienic than the other in adulthood. Hygiene concerns come down to the practices of each adult, as with all genitals.

Circumcision is a hot topic and can have a lot of cultural and religious influences around it, making some people feel abnormal because their penis doesn't look like their peers'. Although some folks have preferences, most do not. As with everything we've discussed about bodies, it's up to each person to decide what level of sensitivity they experience, how they like to be touched, and how they want to embrace their body.

Testicles are the part of the reproductive center that houses sperm, and they are encased in a thin layer of tissue called the *scrotum*.

Now that you have the basics of anatomy, you'll continue to rewrite your sexual narrative by learning how to make friends with your body with the *Going Deeper* exercise at the end of the chapter.

Understanding "Sex" Versus "Gender" for Optimizing Arousal and Connection

When talking about genitals, the term "sex" refers to the genetic expression and appearance of genitals. It's a biological term and what's written on your birth certificate and decided by a healthcare professional or your birthing parents.

"Gender" is the expression of behavior, appearance, and assigned roles society places on a person based on their genitals and societal assumptions. It's a complex cultural concept that has evolved. It is essential to realize that society and culture construct our ideas of gender. Biology can influence gender, but biological sex does not determine one's gender (although exciting new research might reveal something different by the time this book is published). This means that there is a fluidity to gender that doesn't fit into the constraints of a binary expression of "man" or "woman."

Gender is a spectrum, or better yet, more like a 3D graph—up and down, side to side, and even toward and away.

For anyone else who needs it a little more simplified, think about it this way: sex is what's between the legs, and gender is what's between the ears (meaning it's constructed within the mind). Although that's a black-and-white way to think about it, if this is your first time exploring these concepts, it's a good starting point to understand the distinction for now.

Why does this matter for arousal, pleasure, and connection? For so many reasons. However, I can only dip into this topic by focusing on some of the most common reasons I hear from my clients.

Gender can be a helpful way for people to express who they are and how they want the world to see them. It can help folks connect with others who have the same gender identity as they do, and it can help people simplify the process of finding genders they want to spend more time with or pursue sexually or romantically.

However, the concept of gender can also be problematic in a lot of ways. For instance, there is significant societal pressure on cis women or folks socialized as female to be caretakers, people-pleasers, and "polite," causing those folks to overexert themselves for their family or at work while neglecting their own needs and ultimately burn out. Among the many problems this causes, it also significantly impacts sexual arousal and sexual satisfaction, which we'll get into in the next chapter.

Alternatively, society tells kids and adults that it is unacceptable for people socialized as males to express emotions or displays of affection with each other. This causes a lot of cis men and people assigned male at birth (AMAB) to suppress their feelings and create intimacy barriers. Their partners might even be subjected to this harmful belief system, thinking of them as "weak" or "too sensitive" if they cry or have big emotions beyond anger. Large numbers of cis men seek services with sex therapists because when a sexual relationship becomes intimate or requires emotional availability, they often report losing interest in their partner or having difficulty with their erections or sexual satisfaction.

News flash: All humans have emotions, and there's no specific gender that allows some to feel emotions while others cannot. So, if you've ever heard and believed "men don't cry," you've been a victim of harmful social messaging. Everyone's feelings are valid and supported here.

You might not realize that the expectations you have of a partner are related to gender roles even when they don't seem like it. Gender roles can also create tension in same-sex, queer, or polyamorous relationships when partners (sub)consciously are influenced by how someone should behave or think based on their gender.

People struggling with societal expectations around gender often think there's something wrong with them or their bodies when confronting sexual or intimate challenges. The truth is that they're in an oppressive system with cultural pressures on them to be different from what's actually healthy and biologically normal.

Another way that the concept of gender can be harmful is when people don't accept and support the gender a person identifies with. Despite the apparent fact that people need to mind their own business, this is another example of outdated and oppressive belief systems woven into our society that creates long-term effects on non-binary, trans, genderfluid, or queer folks.

Prejudice like this can cause anxiety, trauma, and overwhelming pressure to believe it's unacceptable to be who they are at their core. Expressing oneself sexually and intimately is not the only barrier. Hate crimes and discrimination also cause difficulties with self-esteem, mental well-being, and physical health.

Understanding that gender can have a significant influence on sexual arousal, pleasure, and intimate connection is a vital process in rewriting your sexual narrative. Regardless of your sex or gender, you have been impacted by cultural and societal narratives around gender, even if you're not aware of how. Exploring your thoughts, feelings, and experiences related to gender can help you uncover even more belief systems impacting your sexual arousal and pleasure. Ideally, examining these will also deepen your understanding of those around you and society at large.

You can ask yourself questions like the following and reflect on them or even journal about them:

- What does it mean to me to be a [insert your gender]?
- What are some messages that I understand or believe about [your gender]?
- Do any of those messages or beliefs feel unpleasant when I think about them? Do any of them feel pleasant?
- Do I like the expectations of my gender? If not, why not? If yes, why?
- If you're partnered: What do I think it means to my partner that I'm a [your gender]? What does it mean to me that my partner is a [their gender]? What are my expectations of my partner based on their gender?

Pleasure for Gender Diverse Folks

Most sexual health education lacks sufficient information tailored to folks who exist outside the binary "male-female" concepts. Admittedly, I'm only scratching the surface here myself. Still, it's paramount to decentralize our society's obsession with the binary, non-kinky ("vanilla"), monogamous, and heterosexual concepts of sexual pleasure.

Even if you are cisgender and heterosexual, it's essential to know about other people's experiences. And who knows, if someone close to you begins to embrace a gender beyond the binary, wouldn't you want to feel like you have some foundational understanding that their experience is 100 percent normal?

Just as with cisgender folks, each intersex, trans, or non-binary person can have unique desires and boundaries. If you identify beyond the binary, explore your body with love, give yourself compassion and celebration for the healthy boundaries you want to place around your body, pleasure practices, and sexual experiences. If you're a partner of an intersex, trans, or non-binary person, take into consideration the distinctive experiences around the preferences or differences your partner might have with their genitals.

There can be a lot of emotion attached to the parts of intersex, trans, and non-binary bodies that are involved in sexual play. Certain aspects of their anatomy can be reminders of being born in a body that might not align with what feels right for them. Also, surgery or hormones can cause uncomfortable physical sensations on certain parts of their bodies and genitals. In some circumstances, using particular terms for gender expression and genitals might feel like a trigger for some folks because we've been socialized to think of bodies and gender expression in terms of "feminine" or "masculine," whereas that might not be someone's experience of those concepts at all. Sex acts might also be uncomfortable for some folks because it's been too connected to their biological sex, so they prefer to avoid them.

For instance, one of my clients, a non-binary person assigned male at birth, preferred sexual acts that didn't explicitly involve their penis. They felt conflicted by and uncomfortable with receiving a blow job or providing penetrative sex. Instead, they preferred using a prostate massager while rubbing themselves against a partner to reach orgasm. On the other hand, some folks don't feel the need for certain genitals to define their gender.

If you are not an intersex, trans, or non-binary person, it can be helpful for you to know about this because a partner of yours might be, and getting a brief introduction here can make a world of difference to someone who might share about their sexual or gender identity with you.

Also, as mentioned, it's crucial to get consent to ask or talk to them about their bodies. Just because you don't know about it and are curious doesn't mean you can plow away with questions. They might prefer that you do your own research first or that they need to be more comfortable with you before sharing details about their body and genitals. Our sex-negative culture has attached so much shame to anyone who exists outside of the binary that these can be vulnerable topics to discuss for people who don't identify with binary definitions.

The Anatomy of Arousal and Pleasure

The following areas are notable for arousal and pleasure. This is not the case for everyone and can differ even within the day for someone. Exploring and being curious are the best mindset tools for optimizing your pleasure potential.

The Largest Sex Organ: The Brain

Remember that your sexual arousal system is a lot more accessible and active when the nervous system is well-regulated. Don't limit your pleasure by focusing on the genitals and staying stuck in an activated, stressed, or anxious state.

Off to Find the Mythical Clitoris

The *clitoris* is magical, alright. It's also very real, even though some folks don't know it exists or think it's mythical lore. Despite being able to provide intense pleasure, it's shocking how ignored the clit is in sexual play for folks that have them. That's due mainly to the penis-centered, shame-based sexual health education system.

Recent research has emerged, finding that the clitoris has an average of 10,280 sensitive nerve endings—that's almost triple the amount found in the head of a penis—and highly concentrated in a tiny area of the vulva, which is why it can be so pleasurable (sometimes necessary) to stimulate during play or for sexual arousal.[8]

The structure of the clitoris looks more like a wishbone, with the head at the top of a three-pronged structure. The *clitoral bulbs* can be 3–4 inches in length, and they are located within the body, extending around the vaginal canal. During arousal, the clitoris engorges with blood—just like a penis does, since the bulbs are like the structures within a penis. In Figure 6.4, you can see how a clitoris looks when it's flaccid and how it expands as it becomes erect. Touching the clit in both stages can be highly pleasurable and lead directly to orgasm, or it can be too sensitive to touch. Stimulation around the vulva and inside of the vagina often stimulates the clitoral bulbs, which is why it's critical to learn about what you or your partner likes. Doing this

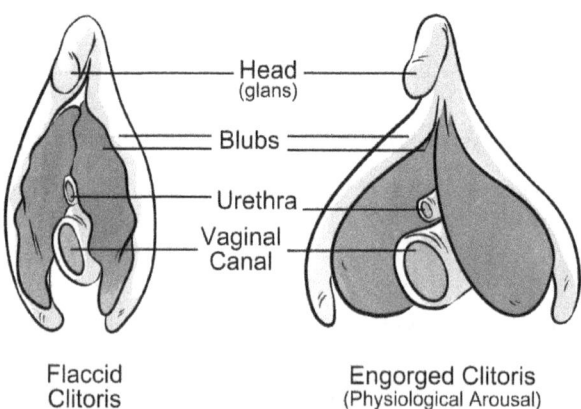

FIGURE 6.4 *Clitoris (internal structure): Flaccid versus engorged comparison.*

would increase the possibilities for arousal and orgasm if that's what you're looking for.

Not all clits are made the same. Just like with vulvas, it's normal for them to be different sizes and to give different ranges of pleasure. Some folks don't like their clit touched directly or with firm pressure, while others need firm pressure for pleasure optimization. Everyone is different and can change as arousal increases.

Despite what most people think, orgasm from vaginal penetration alone only occurs in about 18 percent of vulva owners.[9] That means that most vulvas need clitoral stimulation if they want to achieve an orgasm. However, most heterosexual couples and cis women expect the female partner to be able to achieve pleasure and orgasm just from penile penetration.

Biology and the development of genitals in a fetus can help you understand why those beliefs are highly problematic.

Within the first two months of gestation, the fetus begins to develop its genitals. Before that, the genital structures looked the same as in the initial stage in Figure 6.5 (the center image). Once the biological sex starts to develop,

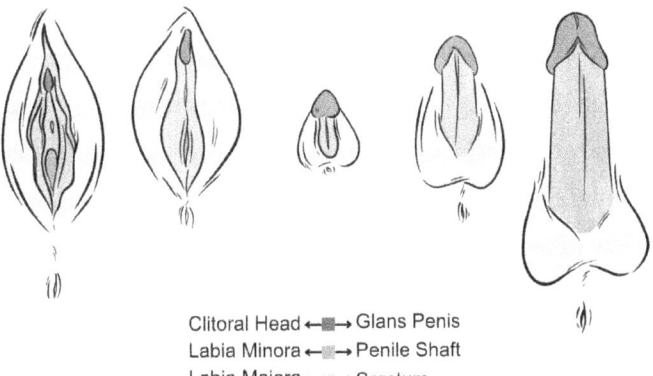

Clitoral Head ←■→ Glans Penis
Labia Minora ←■→ Penile Shaft
Labia Majora ← →Scrotum

FIGURE 6.5 *External genitalia development in utero. Starts at the indifferent stage (center) and grows differentially into a clitoris (left) or penis (right). Fully formed by 17–18 weeks.*

in most cases, the structures grow into either a penis or a vulva, as you see in the other stages of Figure 6.5.

Despite differences in appearance or location, most bodies have the same genital parts even if they're organized in different places. These are called "homologous structures." For instance, the head of the penis and the shaft are the structures of the clitoral head and bulbs. The scrotum on a body born with a penis is the same skin structure as the outer lips of the vulva once it develops in utero.

The reason this is important is that our culture has prioritized penis-in-vagina (PIV) sex and largely ignored the importance of clitoral stimulation, focusing primarily on the pleasure of the penis. In PIV sex, the penis head (which has the most pleasurable nerve endings) and shaft receive stimulation until the person with a penis reaches orgasm. However, the vaginal opening does not have nearly enough pleasurable sensitive nerve endings for the stimulation to equal that of the penis. For it to be close to the same, the clitoris needs just as much attention as the penis receives.

Imagine if we reversed the focus of stimulation on the structures—that a cisgender heterosexual couple stimulated the cis woman's parts with the man's parts using the homologous structures as in PIV sex. The cis man rubs his scrotum and shaft on his partner's clitoris until she reaches orgasm, and then they wonder why he didn't come. It might feel pleasurable enough for him, but it's not enough to get him to orgasm. It seems silly to think of it this way, but that's what we're doing when we prioritize PIV sex without clitoral stimulation.

Ignoring the clit and thinking penetration alone should be sufficient is one of the main reasons there's an "orgasm gap" between cis women and their male partners. In heterosexual sex, about 91 percent of men reported having an orgasm, while women reported only 39 percent.[10] The critical takeaway is (if you or your partner has a clitoris): include the clit into the mix, and all parties may have much more arousal, pleasure, and orgasm.

"G-Spot"

Inside the vaginal canal, about 1–2 inches toward the top front wall, is an area that is commonly called the *G-spot*. The existence of the G-spot is controversial.[11] Some people don't notice a difference in sensation when stimulating this area, some dislike stimulation in that area, and others report significantly pleasurable sensitivity and that it can contribute to ejaculation in bodies with vaginas.

Furthermore, sensitizing this spot could take some time, so it might need continual and direct stimulation before it becomes pleasurable. You can play around with it to learn what works. Your experience is your own; if you (or your partner) love to be stimulated there, fantastic! If you don't feel anything (or don't like it) but think you should because that's what media, porn, or partners have told you is "normal," remember that sexual empowerment comes from finding what works for you and tossing out belief systems that make you think there's something wrong with you (or your partner).

Chest of Treasure

Considered secondary sex characteristics, the *breasts* and *chest* on many bodies can enhance arousal and pleasure. Breasts can be stimulated in a variety of ways to create pleasure, including the *nipples* and *areola* (the area around the nipple).

Moms or birthing parents who are breastfeeding or have kids may have a difficult time incorporating their breasts into sexual play since the primary role of their breasts is a feed factory. It can take some time, if ever, for someone to reclaim pleasure after this. Also, getting "touched out" is a real thing—parents report feeling overstimulated by the touching requirements kids have, especially the breastfeeding parent. So, touching breasts for sexual arousal or pleasure with their partners can be too much for them, and the sexual arousal system often turns off or is hard to activate. That's where the Arousal Architecture®can be used (more on that soon)!

Family Jewels

The *testicles* and *scrotum* can be highly pleasurable areas. Many people do not like a lot of pressure or firm touch since these parts are delicate and can be easily hurt. Others who are kinky and into "cock-and-ball torture" like a lot of pain there.

Incorporating touch or grip on or around the scrotum or testicles with sexual play like oral, anal, or manual sex can profoundly enhance pleasure for the penis owner. Playing with this area can also be a great way to pivot from focusing on the penis if you want to prolong orgasm, remove pressure or focus on an erect penis, or use it as a precursor to touching the penis directly.

Butt Stuff

Anal stimulation is something I highly recommend for almost everyone. The *anus* has a lot of pleasurable nerve endings around it. It can enhance sexual play by stroking the skin tissue, licking the area ("rimming"), or inserting fingers or hands ("fisting"), toys, or penises. When inserting anything in the anus, make sure to use lots of lube and reapply regularly; start by inserting slowly; communicate effectively about speed, pressure, and intensity; and always use something with a flare or base to avoid a trip to the emergency room to get it removed. There are many more tips for successful anal play, but these are some basics!

The *anus* and *prostate* in cis men or bodies born with penises can be overlooked pleasure centers, especially by heterosexual cis men, because society has told them that this area is "only for gay men." This belief couldn't be further from the truth. I mean, think about it—when male DNA was developing in a fetus, it didn't decide only to form sensitive nerve endings in the bodies of gay babies.

The stigma around cis men enjoying anal pleasure is another societal construct. If you or your partner believes otherwise, one or both of you are missing out on a lot of fun. Folks with prostates who stimulate them during sexual play say that it's much more enjoyable than ignoring it. "Pegging" is all the rage in many enlightened circles. It refers to when a partner without a penis (e.g., cis woman, non-binary person) wears a strap-on with a dildo and inserts it into their partner's anus. It can be very erotic, intensely pleasurable (especially if the inserting partner creates stimulation on their genitals as well, such as with a vibrator on their clit, at the same time), and intimately bonding.

That's my public service announcement for folks who have never considered anal play. I hope you'll rethink how much more pleasure you can have if you release the belief systems suppressing your pleasure—you can take it or leave it!

Also, *spanking* the tushie can be a glorious experience if you or your partner are into it, and there's actually a physiological explanation for why (it's not necessarily because you're a little kinky). Sensitive and arousing nerves run from the space between the top of the thigh and the butt cheek, which I like to call the "thut" (thigh and butt). Spanking doesn't have to be about intensity, pain, or even punishment (although if that's your thing, I totally get it!). Even lightly or rhythmically tapping this area can soothe the nervous system and increase arousal.

Literally Anywhere

Your entire body can be an erogenous zone, especially if you include your brain to create conditions for desire and safety.[12] You just need to be willing to explore and wire your pleasure pathways for a focus beyond genitals, too.

Not all places feel good to everyone. Sometimes, those pleasure places might change depending on your mood, phase of the menstrual cycle, or level of arousal. Self-exploration and effective communication about this are crucial when bringing your whole body into play.

Many cis women express frustration to me about how their heterosexual partners constantly neglect other parts of their bodies and go straight for their breasts or vulvas. Also, cis men and folks with penises have shared that they feel limited with their sexual expression because it's mainly focused on their penis. When you don't incorporate all your body or your partner's body (including the brain) into sexual play, you're narrowing your ability to access arousal, pleasure, and orgasm. If that feels like an uncomfortable suggestion—fear not! You'll get to practice and learn to overcome discomfort more easily soon.

Hitting That Peak: Orgasms

Although one of my primary points in this book is about creating pleasure and reducing pressure or focusing on orgasm, orgasms are likely going to be a part of your experience. We love them, but we want to reduce the pressure and enhance overall well-being since orgasms can have fantastic health benefits, and limited orgasms are associated with depression.[13]

There are anecdotal concepts and some conflicting science about the different types of orgasms. I've heard of folks having clitoral, vaginal, penile, anal, nipple, whole body, energetic, "G-spot," cervical, and ejaculatory orgasms. I wish I could dive deep into each of these, but there's much to say (I go more in-depth on my website, socials, and YouTube if you want to check them out). Still, the point I want to make here is that your body can have the potential for a lot of different kinds of pleasure and sensations during sexual play that can lead to a variety of orgasmic experiences.

I want to caution you against using this information to beat yourself up if you have difficulty with orgasm at the moment. Don't use this as a measuring stick—you just need to put into practice the skills we've discussed or get the right kind of professional support to help you on your journey!

Using the tools in this book can help you create a path toward many types of orgasms because two of the most critical factors in achieving orgasm are the right mindset and tools to keep you present and directed toward pleasure.

The Science of Arousal and Pleasure

Numerous foundational models for sexual arousal have been important jumping-off points for improving sexual satisfaction and relationships. Now, we'll explore some of those concepts as well as a few of my favorite modernized ones so that you have the most well-rounded, science-informed understanding of what's going on with your mind and body when it comes to sex, especially if you've been struggling with arousal, pleasure, and intimacy.

We'll explore the basic definitions of sexual arousal functioning, sexual response cycle models, and why it's crucial to know about "spontaneous desire" versus "responsive desire." Dr. Emily Nagoski's *Come as You Are* and *Come Together* are pivotal books in helping people and couples understand crucial sexual science to improve their sex lives and relationships.[14] I highly recommend reading those for a deep dive—they'll blow your mind. In this book, I'm barely touching on the depth of that inspiring science she masterfully explains to provide you with an overview and a system to apply it all to (the Arousal Architecture®).

Sexual Health Definitions

The following are definitions of sexual health and wellness that we all should have been taught but probably weren't, at least not correctly for most.

Desire and Arousal

Although "sex drive" is frequently used to describe "sexual arousal" or "desire," it's not entirely accurate. Let's get clear about what these terms mean.

Sexual desire is what happens in the mind (the thoughts, ideas, or fantasies) that you have about sex that can contribute to sexual arousal, but not always. It's also influenced by a person's psychological state or relational interactions, such as mental health or connection with a partner. This is the process that occurs when you feel motivated psychologically to seek out a sexual experience, and many refer to it as a *libido*.

Sexual arousal is the physiological response and changes that occur in the body, such as lubrication or erection. It's created by sexual contact or by other erotic stimulations (e.g., fantasies, dreams, odors, or objects). This process starts as the brain and body receive input or stimulation and send messages through the central nervous system to the rest of the body, mainly the genitals.[15]

Even though it seems like *arousal* and *desire* would occur at the same time, you can have sexual desire but not physiological arousal. Alternatively, you can be physically aroused but not have a desire to express yourself sexually or even know why you feel aroused. Say what!?

This mind-blowing phenomenon is called "arousal non-concordance," and although not new to sexology, it is still very foreign to the everyday person.

A myth I love busting is the idea that penises must be erect if they're aroused, and if they're not erect, they must not be aroused or have sexual desire. Understanding that this can happen removes pressure on penis owners to "perform" (via an erection) as an expression of their desire or alleviate concerns of their partners that something is "wrong," such as with Jason.

Case Study: Jason (he/him)

One of my bisexual male clients expressed concern that his partner didn't desire him because when they were kissing and touching each other, he didn't feel him get hard. This experience created a spiral of anxiety and disconnection because Jason knew that his penis always became erect whenever he had a desire for his partners. After explaining to him that desire and sexual arousal don't always coincide, he felt relieved. It inspired a conversation between them, and Jason's partner confirmed that he sincerely desired him and that, on occasion, his penis doesn't become erect as quickly as other times.

Another point of interest around *arousal non-concordance* is from a study that compared male and female arousal states when watching porn. Most of the men knew when they were aroused. Conversely, the women did not always know when they were aroused.[16]

What does it mean for you? It could mean that you might want to be aroused, but your body isn't there yet. It's also possible that you're physiologically aroused, and you might not notice it.

The point is that your mind can be very influential when you create meaning about how your body is reacting, which can be a common struggle for people dealing with sexual challenges like pain or anxiety.

What can you do about it? Use the tools you've been building, such as redirecting your thoughts when you begin spiraling or thinking too hard about what's happening. You can refocus back on neutral sensations or experiences, especially when having sex. The heavy emphasis on these tools early in this book helps you build up to using them when thinking, talking about, or having sex.

Does It "Take Long" to Get Aroused?
You Might Have Responsive Desire

Dr. Rosemary Basson developed the "Non-Linear Sexual Response Cycle," a paradigm-shifting concept which helped paved the pathway to understanding the difference between "responsive desire" and "spontaneous desire."[17] Although the concepts were initially applied to the experience of cis women, I've seen all genders relate to it.

Spontaneous desire is what most people are used to when they think about being turned on—it happens "naturally" or spontaneously when you see or think about a person or situation that's typically arousing to you. The desire comes from anticipating pleasure (with yourself or with others).[18] For someone with spontaneous desire, engaging in sexual stimulation after arousal usually increases arousal and leads to orgasm.

For some people, they can be aroused and stay aroused through sexual stimulation until orgasm. Usually, folks who have spontaneous desire also relate to the linear experience of sexual response, as illustrated in Figure 6.6.[19]

Responsive desire refers to the experience people have when their sexual desire or arousal needs more than exposure to sexual stimuli. Context, intimacy, the right mindset, or pleasantly sufficient physical stimulation are some of the stimuli that someone with responsive desire might need before they can be in the mood for sexual play or even before they feel the physiological sexual arousal response (e.g., erection, lubrication, or pleasant tingles). Their desire is in response to pleasure, whether that's emotional, sexual, or even joyful experiences.[20] Folks with responsive desire usually relate more to a non-linear cycle, such as Basson's illustrated in Figure 6.7, instead of the linear model.

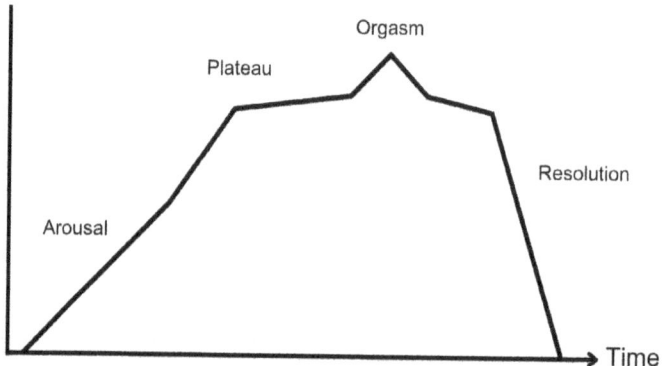

FIGURE 6.6 *Linear model of sexual arousal with physiological stages. Adapted from Masters and Johnson,* Human Sexual Response.

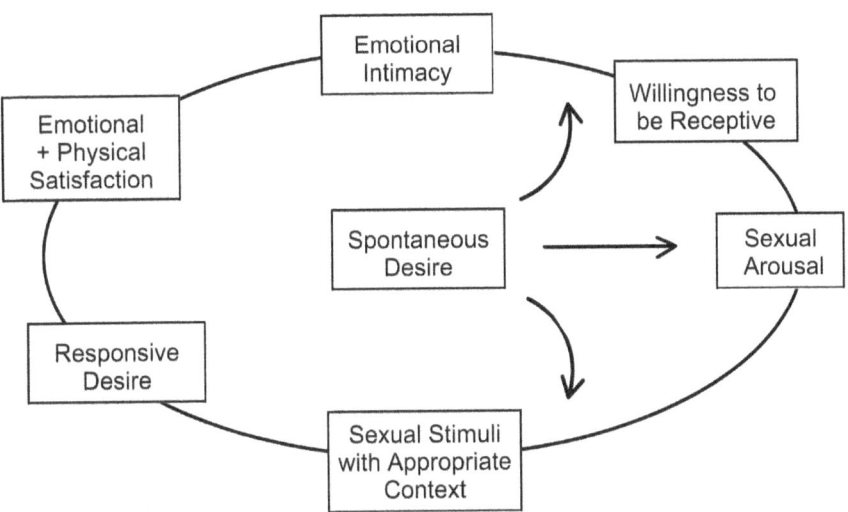

FIGURE 6.7 *Non-Linear Sexual Response Cycle. A cyclical nature of sexual arousal, response, desire, and emotional intimacy within particular contexts. Adapted from Basson, "The New Female," 51–65.*

Like the linear model, in the non-linear sexual response cycle, sexual stimuli *can* be the entry point for someone with a responsive desire to engage in sexual play. Then, once they are aroused or engaging in the play, instead of moving "easily" toward heightened arousal and then orgasm with sufficient stimulation (as with the linear model), there are a lot of other factors that keep someone engaged with and aroused by the sexual experience. These motivating factors might be "non-sexual" rewards like a desire for intimacy or closeness, feeling desired or validated, or seeking relaxation.

In contrast to an upward straight trajectory like the linear model, the non-linear cycle represents a sexual response more like a positive feedback loop: multiple needs and desires beyond sexual stimulation motivate someone to engage in the sexual experience, going around the cycle feeding on the other motivators. If one or more factors become problematic or change during sexual play (e.g., if someone no longer feels relaxed or connected to their partner), their sexual arousal can wane. Their interest in sexual play can stop altogether.

This model and my clients' experiences were the inspiration for creating the Arousal Architecture®. I heard from so many clients that they thought there was something wrong with them because their arousal didn't respond as it "should" or how it did in the past. Folks with responsive arousal systems needed a new way to look at their arousal system. Thanks to Basson's work and the Arousal Architecture®, they now have that, along with a step-by-step process (this book), to find confidence in seeking their unique arousal needs.

The "Dual Control Model of Sexual Response," developed by Dr. John Bancroft and Dr. Erick Janssen, helps us understand how we move toward and away from sexual experiences.[21] Dr. Emily Nagoski popularized the Dual Control Model concept of "brakes" and "accelerators" in her book *Come as You Are*, explaining that sexual desire is like being in a car and that something happens that either moves you toward sexual play or keeps you from moving toward it.[22]

I love this, *and* if we're going with the car metaphor, what if your car doesn't even have gas or you don't even know how to get on the metaphorical road of the Non-Linear Sexual Response Cycle? When you've had anxiety, sexual pain, or other challenges with sex that keep you from easy access to arousal or aversion to sexual stimuli you might need an expanded representation of these models.

Think of your new Expanded Non-Linear Sexual Response Cycle like a racetrack for sexual play—a Sexy Time Track. On that track, some aspects get you on the road, keep you going, block your focus, and take you totally off track. Figure 6.8 provides a visual example of this concept, which has helped my clients conceptualize this.

On your Sexy Time Track, when you have dealt with sexual challenges or outdated belief systems, you might experience the following:

- *On-ramps* are the behaviors, thoughts, and feelings you enjoy, which keep you present and create space for arousal. They inspire motivations

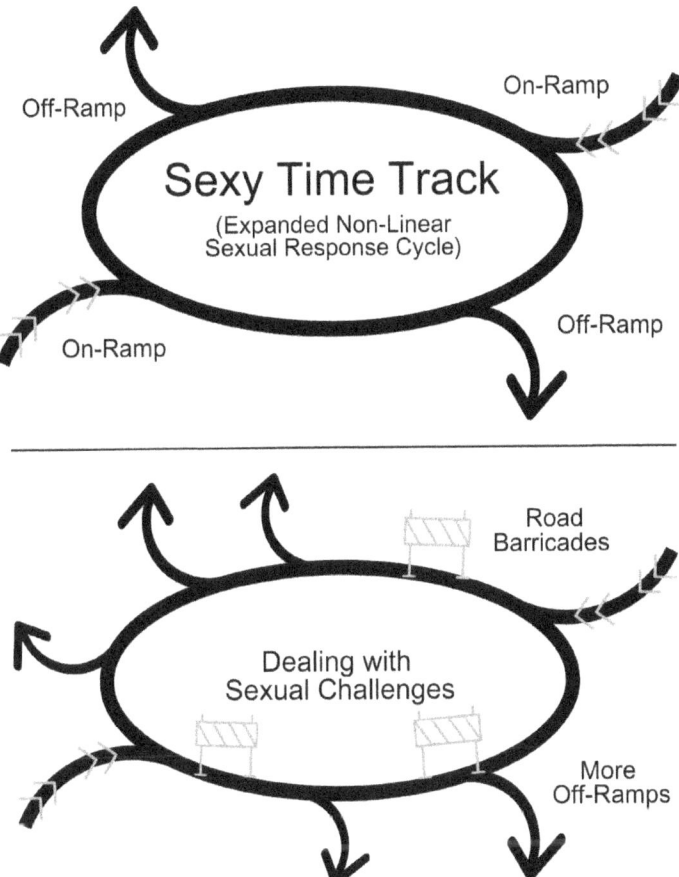

FIGURE 6.8 *Expanded Non-Linear Sexual Response Cycle (Sexy Time Track) and a representation of sexual challenges within the cycle demonstrated by road barricades and increased off-ramps.*

toward sex and arousal. This is similar to "accelerators," except that they also help you arrive at the track before even considering arousal or engaging with sexual stimuli.

- *Off-ramps* can be seen as the judgment, criticism, doubt, and distractions that can easily steer you away from arousal. They're the detours that take you off the main road.

- *Road barricades* are the barriers preventing you from accessing arousal and directing your attention to distracting experiences (just like what you'd see on the road where there is construction and traffic redirection). These are like the "brakes," except that they can even block you from getting to the Sexy Time Track entirely by focusing on "non-intimate" stimulation outside of sexual contexts such as "To Do" lists, overworking, or perfectionism.

Using these models and all the work you've been doing so far in this book can help you in so many ways. Here are examples of how they integrate in a cohesive system:

- You're learning to identify the outdated belief systems around sex and the impact of those beliefs (which are like barricades and off-ramps).

- You've developed skills to regulate your nervous system to help remove barriers from the track. You can also use these tools, along with stimulation you find pleasurable, to "fuel up" so you maintain interest and excitement, create on-ramps, and stay as presently on the track as possible instead of easily getting distracted and finding yourself on an off-ramp.

- The mindset work and new sexual narratives we've explored have helped you create a global positioning system (GPS) in your car that keeps you focused on where you're going and helps redirect you if you happen to take an off-ramp.

- Using compassion and growth-oriented language maintains a healthy way of talking to yourself and others when you encounter barricades and need to pivot or replan your way around the Sexy Time Track.

The Arousal Architecture® will provide even more specific and tangible ideas to help you solidify the confidence you have in maintaining an exciting and rewarding sexual response cycle.

The Myth of "Foreplay"

It's time for some more myth-busting! Another misconception is a thing called "foreplay"—maybe you've heard of it? Even as a sex therapist, I used the term "foreplay" incorrectly for an embarrassingly long time.

Referring to "everything before penetration" as "foreplay" keeps us stuck and limits possibilities for pleasure. Not to mention, it reinforces the concept that PIV is the only "real sex" and sets up some unhealthy expectations.

I dig deeply into this in my coaching and psychotherapy programs with clients. Even though we're just dipping our toes in, you can still benefit greatly from simply suspending belief with me (at least while you're reading this book) that all kinds of activities can be "sex." Flirting can be sex. Kissing can be sex. Going for a walk in the park solo or with a partner can be a part of your sexual on-ramp.

One of my favorite YouTube shorts is a video by Jeff Guenther (a.k.a. @therapyjeff), where he wonderfully exclaims that your next sexual experience happens as soon as the present one ends. He doesn't mean you're having sex all the time. Instead, it means that the possibilities for sexual satisfaction don't have to be limited to one kind of (*cough* heteronormative) sex act.[23]

Tossing out the concept that foreplay exists will reduce pressure and offer opportunities to create more pleasure and satisfaction. You'll learn more about how to make all activities contribute to your sexual arousal and experience using the Arousal Architecture® soon.

Sexual Pleasure Paradigm Shift

The paradigm around what is "normal" or "real" sex is born from the oppressive systems of sex-negative messaging, heteronormativity, and misogyny (such as with penis-focused pleasure). I'm not against giving penises pleasure, don't get me wrong! Instead, it's necessary to look at why most people believe that PIV sex is the "Holy Grail" of sexual acts and consider how it's limiting everyone's pleasure potential, even penis-owners.

Exploring these belief systems and simply acknowledging that they've been feeding you lies about what "normal" is can help you reclaim sexual power no matter what gender you are. PIV sex can be great; I get it. But so much more pleasure and satisfaction can be unlocked in bodies when you consider shifting your understanding from your current perspective to a new one.

The typical paradigm for sexual pleasure preferences looks a lot like a pyramid with PIV sex or penetration at the top and all other sexual play below that, making it seem like those other activities are second best or only precursors to achieve the "best" option. This concept is just like you probably learned about in grade school, framing sexual practices as getting to certain "bases."

Instead, think about sexual activities as a spectrum. No particular sexual activity should be prioritized over others as the best or most important act. This isn't to say that they are all equal in levels of pleasure. Indeed, some sex acts can objectively feel more pleasurable for you or your partner. The aim is to recognize that some people feel more pleasure with some acts and others with other activities. Most importantly, if there *is* a difference within a partnership, both partners' preferences need to be equitably prioritized in sexual play. Utilizing this paradigm shift doesn't mean that every single time you're sexual with a partner, you must include everyone's interests; instead, it's balanced across the span of the relationship.

Figure 6.9 provides some examples to conceptualize a Spectrum of Sexual Play. You can see that Partner A prefers sensual touching, flirting, and banter the most. In contrast, Partner B finds PIV penetration and receiving oral sex the most pleasurable. They both enjoy manual sex and kissing about the same. Neither's preferences are better or more "normal," just different. A healthy sexual dynamic for these two would be one where they were engaging in flirting and sensual touching about the same amount as various types of penetration, for example.

You could write out your own spectrum and share it with a partner or have it for yourself to explore the various ways you enjoy and prioritize certain

YOUR BODY

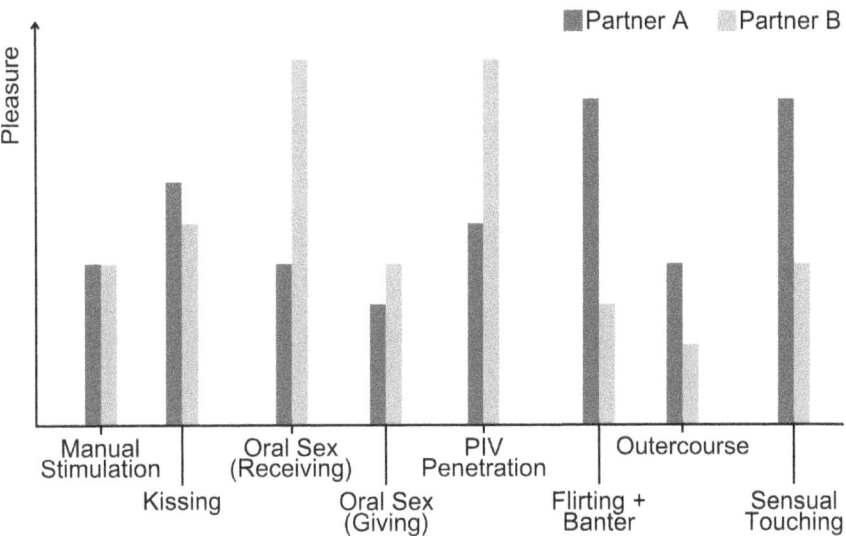

FIGURE 6.9 *Comparison between Partner A's and Partner B's interests in activities on the Spectrum of Sexual Play.*

self-pleasure activities. Comparing yours (non-judgmentally) with your partner's could help you find activities you both enjoy. By doing so, you might also learn that one person's experience of pleasure is getting more prioritized over the other. This is not to say that one person is a bad or selfish sexual partner if you realize this. Being the compassionate scientist you are, uncovering this data can help inform decisions moving forward. Engaging in this paradigm shift optimizes pleasure, breaks the stigma that only certain kinds of acts are "sex," and reduces pressure to perform. All these can be critical factors in rewriting your sexual narrative when using the Arousal Architecture® which we'll get into next!

Pleasure Gems

- Becoming familiar with your body and the parts of others' bodies is crucial for enhancing pleasure and confidence.

- Reconsider ideas around gender and expectations so that you feel more empowered in your sexual narrative.

- Your entire body (and that of a partner's) can be an erotic zone. Explore the areas that seem exciting to you and learn what doesn't.

- The Dual Control Model, Non-Linear Female Sexual Response Cycle, and your new Expanded Non-Linear Model (the Sexy Time Track) help folks understand that spontaneous desire isn't the only way people can get aroused.

- Using the concepts and interventions you've learned so far can help you identify metaphorical on-ramps, off-ramps, and barricades that can either enhance your sexual arousal or keep you from staying in a satisfying sexual response cycle.

- Busting the myth of foreplay and creating a Sexual Pleasure Paradigm Shift can help you optimize possibilities for arousal and pleasure.

Exercises

Quick Win!

Build a Pleasurable Connection Beyond Your Genitals

The goal is to wire pleasurable sensations to other areas of your body that you might not realize can be woven into the erotic map of your body. Spend two to three minutes daily with this exercise for a week.

1. Start with one hand on your pelvic area or genitals and notice the sensations that come up. If you experience mostly unpleasant sensations while doing this, notice what arises, acknowledge it, increase compassion for yourself, and regulate your nervous system, or redirect your attention back to a neutral sensation in or around

the area, if possible, or anywhere else in your body if you can't locate neutral sensations at that moment.

2. Use your other hand to touch other body parts, such as your neck, abdomen, arms, or feet. Try different types of touch, such as stroking your hand along that part of your body or simply keeping your hand placed there.

3. Notice the pleasant sensations that come up.

This can be a beneficial exercise for people with physically painful sex, pelvic pain, erectile variability, and difficulty with orgasm. It's also helpful if you tend to focus primarily on traditional genital stimulation to achieve sexual pleasure, helping you expand possibilities for pleasure.

Going Deeper

Mirror Exercise

This exercise will help you become better acquainted with your genitals. It might initially feel uncomfortable, so remember to be kind to yourself and use your nervous system regulation techniques to bring your body and mind to a mostly neutral experience. Keep an eye out for any pleasant moment! This practice can be very powerful especially if you tend to avoid touching your genitals.

1. Get a mirror that you can explore your genitals with comfortably.
2. Locate the anatomical parts and common pleasure centers on your genitals.
3. You can use the figures in this chapter to guide you.
4. If you're feeling overwhelmed with unpleasant sensations, use the tools and interventions we've discussed so far to help you regulate and reach mostly neutral.

Breathe Out Anxiety, Breathe In Arousal

This exercise has three stages. You can make it as spicy or mild as you want. It will help you rewire your nervous system's response to experiences that typically activate discomfort or aversion.

1. Write a list of three sensual touch or visual experiences, listing them in order of "least distressing" to "most distressing."
2. In the first stage, you'll start with the least distressing activity, and as you engage in it, notice any unpleasant sensations, thoughts, or feelings that arise.
3. Utilize the tools and practices we've discussed (acknowledge, create compassion, and regulate using mindfulness or somatic interventions that have worked well for you so far). Your primary aim is to seek neutral or pleasant sensations.
4. Continue to engage in this activity until you notice mostly neutral sensations, thoughts, or feelings.
5. Once you feel *mostly* neutral, move on to the next distressing activity and repeat the process for the second and third stages.

I've included a list of ideas or suggestions you could try in this exercise.

- Look at your body fully clothed in the mirror. Then, look at your body in your underwear. Finally, look at your body naked in the mirror.
- Place your hand over your genitals or breasts over your clothes. Then, place your hand over your genitals or breasts over your underwear. Finally, place your hand over your genitals or breasts with skin-to-skin contact.
- Stroke parts of your body that are not your genitals or breasts, then stroke around your genitals or breasts, but do not touch directly on

your genitals or nipples. Finally, stroke, caress, and rub your genitals or around your nipples or breasts.

Doing this or finding alternatives that work for you empowers you to take control and develop autonomy over your sexual narrative.

Make a Sexual Pleasure Paradigm Shift

The goal of this exercise is to create a perspective shift around how you view and prioritize certain sexual activities. You'll do this by creating your Spectrum of Sexual Play.

1. First, list out all the options of sexual play that you have done or would like to do. This can be your "Sexual Menu." Although almost anything can be considered part of sexual play, for now, focus on explicitly sexual, intimate, and sensual behaviors or activities.

2. Next to each item on your list, rate on a scale from 1 to 10 how much you enjoy that activity, where 1 is "a little bit" and 10 is "this is my favorite thing!" You can have the same rating for multiple activities.

3. If you're a visual person, you could place them along the spectrum, as in Figure 6.9, without putting them in any particular order. You can make the heights of the lines longer to indicate a higher pleasure ranking.

4. If you have a partner, ask your partner to make their own with you and then share them. Have an objective and compassionate conversation about what shifts you would like to make to your current sexual practices. The conversation interventions in Part 4 can help if you need extra support.

7

Your Energy
Holistic Sexual Wellness

Regardless of your belief system around spirituality or energetics (such as experiencing something you can't really put into exact words, but you know it's happening), there is an aspect of our lives that impacts sexual satisfaction that many folks often overlook. It's what I'm calling "Energy" in this book since it's the least controversial and most scientifically informed way to describe this part of our sexualities. Other folks call this part of themselves their psyche, spirit, soul, or emotional body. Whatever you call it, I'm here for it and celebrate it!

Incorporating the whole person into the transformation is necessary. We can't just look at our sex lives.

Sex can be a barometer of sorts. It might be the first indicator that something in your life is not running smoothly. Sexual arousal is a "luxury system," so if your life requires a lot of energy and resources to manage daily tasks or stressors, then there might not be much remaining for sexual arousal.

Within this chapter, I'll identify some of the most common challenges that can impact your overall sense of who you are and what's going on in life beyond sex. We'll explore how personal passion or a sense of purpose can influence how sexual you want to be. Additionally, I'll highlight struggles that people often have that seem unrelated to their sex lives. Eventually, they realize there's a much more significant impact than they thought. Understanding this and reflecting on your own life can help you determine if you need to change those parts of your life. You also might experience validation as you learn how external influences can shape your experiences as a sexual human.

Another aspect of energy to explore is what makes you want to avoid sex or contribute to the Sexual Aversion Cycle by investigating social, cultural, or relational components. These areas might offer insight into why sexual challenges and experiences are about more than "simply" erection or arousal issues.

Don't worry; I won't leave you in dismay, though! I'll guide you through how to find what energetically motivates you toward sex and how to amplify it.

What Makes You Avoid Sex?

There can be many reasons seemingly unrelated to sex that will be important to explore if sex and arousal have ever felt problematic. The first step is identifying if you (sub)consciously avoid sex. Do any of the following resonate with you?

- Getting on your iPad or Kindle in bed instead of taking time to connect with your partner.
- Creating "busy work" until you're too tired or your schedule is too packed, so you "don't have time" for sex.
- Feeling relieved when you or your partner is menstruating or out of town for a few days, meaning sex isn't required of you.
- Choosing not to have sex because you're upset or annoyed with your partner, even though part of you wants sex.

If so, you might be (unknowingly) using these tactics to keep the Sexual Aversion Cycle active. Doing these things doesn't mean there's anything wrong with you. It just means that it's essential to explore what's happening energetically for you that's contributing to sexual avoidance.

Even if you don't avoid sex, being aware of these hurdles can help you prevent them in the future. Furthermore, you can identify if you might miss opportunities to expand your arousal potential.

How Psychological and External Forces Feed the Sexual Aversion Cycle

I don't know what's wrong with me.

When my partner hugs me and starts to kiss me, my body tightens up. I either have no thoughts at all, and I feel frozen, or my mind is racing with all of the possible ways I can get out of having sex.

Then I feel sooo bad. He's amazing, and I love him, but I just can't get myself in the mood.

Am I just not attracted to him anymore? Did we lose our spark?

I feel so worried and hopeless about what this means. Am I broken?

The above was a conversation I had in a Consultation Call with someone wanting to work with me due to their "lack of arousal and interest in sex." And it's something I've heard in some fashion many times each year since 2006 when I started in the field of human sexuality.

They are also similar to thoughts I had myself when struggling with unwanted sexual pain. Maybe it resonates with you, too?

This couple had tried intimacy workshops, date nights, and traditional couples therapy. Nothing was working long-term. After we explored areas of their lives that were contributing to the energetic tension of their sexual dissatisfaction beyond the act of sex, they were able to interrupt the Sexual Aversion Cycle and create a new sexual narrative for their relationship.

The sexual arousal system is more like a reward system: the better sex feels (emotionally, physically, and energetically), the more you want it. However, the more sex or intimacy causes discomfort or pain, the more you withdraw and run in the other direction. It's like expecting yourself to be excited to go to a family gathering that always ends with Auntie criticizing your hair and bringing up what a disappointment she thinks everyone is. How could you expect to get excited about the next family birthday party?

As you attempt to engage in unpleasant sexual situations without effective interventions to interrupt the pattern, it becomes a vicious cycle—and goodbye sexual arousal.

This aversion pattern doesn't happen because you want it to. Like most of my clients, you probably *want to want* sex, but your body isn't aligned with your mind's desire for a satisfying sex life. From the previous chapters, you now know that this can happen because of a protective response and because your brain is wired to allocate resources to survival or other valuable situations that bring you more pleasure and less-demanding experiences like binge-watching the latest Netflix show, spending time with friends, or scrolling on social media.

However, life circumstances, relationship issues, or cultural barriers can also contribute to how you feel about yourself, your body, and your sex life from a larger perspective. In that case, they also might be interjecting their influences in ways you don't even realize—they can be very sneaky!

You're Not Broken—The System Is

Social and cultural messages create deep-rooted beliefs about sex that often feel like facts. In reality, these are learned responses, as we discussed in Part 1. You now have the tools to start rewriting those that no longer serve you.

However, other socio-cultural aspects of life can influence your sexual wellness. Many people internalize these influences, believing they're "bad" at sex or "just not a sexual person." While there are folks who don't identify as sexual people, such as asexual folks, others think they're not sexual due to these external forces. If that resonates with you, I'm here to tell you that it's not that you're not good at sex. Or that you're "just not sexual." You're not broken; the system you learned about sex from is.

Think about the sex education you had, if any. If it was like mine, it was "sex-negative," providing limited, fear-based information. Most sex education is abstinence-only, focusing on preventing sex rather than making informed, empowered choices about health. Despite their intent, these programs didn't stop teens from having sex or reduce teen pregnancies; instead, they led to higher health issues, including teen pregnancies.[1]

Being "sex-positive" means reducing shame about sexual practices and orientation, providing accurate information, and emphasizing safer sex practices. It also involves teaching about pleasure-oriented practices like using lube and communicating boundaries and desires, which is seen as a fundamental human right in many other countries but not in the United States.[2] Coincidentally, the United States has higher rates of unwanted teen pregnancies and sexually transmitted infections.[3]

It's mind-blowing to think we're expected to have good sex and relationships, given what we were taught. Recognizing where and how you learned about sex is crucial to understanding why you believe what you believe about sex, especially subconsciously. If you think your sex life could be better, knowing where and how you learned about sex is vital to unlocking arousal-stifling belief systems.

The "energy" of what we learn creates problems—belief systems are energy, and social influence creates energy. These problematic belief systems result in common misconceptions and messages around sex, such as:

- Sexual desire is something you have or don't have. If you don't have sex often enough or in the right way, something is wrong with you.
- Successful sex is related to reaching orgasm, ensuring your partner has their ideal experience, and proving you're enjoying yourself.

- Sex = penis-in-vagina intercourse; everything else is less valuable.

- There is a "right" way to be sexy: not too sexual, not too prudish, not silly or lighthearted.

- If your partner knows you well enough or is genuinely into you, they should know what works for you and are responsible for your sexual satisfaction.

Likely, most sources you've been exposed to around sex, your body, intimacy, or relationships don't provide a realistic portrayal of everyday, sometimes awkward, sometimes unexciting sex. They also probably don't demonstrate healthy communication about boundaries, pleasure-based needs, or enthusiastic consent.

So, how are you expected to have the skills to feel comfortable in your body, prioritize pleasure, and communicate effectively with sexual partners?

Understanding these socio-cultural aspects can help you identify and overcome beliefs that hinder your sexual wellness.

Discrimination and Sex: The Impact of Racism, Oppression, and Prejudice

This section will briefly explore intersectional complexities that could impact sexuality and intimacy. Even though the following is an oversimplified snapshot of how people dealing with oppression navigate life, I aim to shed light on experiences that could impact sexual wellness and intimate connection.

I belong to a few communities that experience oppression (being a woman, queer, and having an invisible disability), and I know the toll oppression wreaks on my nervous system and sex life. There are many communities in which I will never fully understand the experiences of oppression they've had to deal with. Those experiences and the following topics could be in their own library wing. Still, since it's beyond the scope of this book to dive deeper, I hope it provides enough validation and context for those facing oppression and sexual challenges. As this is not meant to be exhaustive, at the back of the book you'll find additional resources, including people of color scholars, researchers, and resources that can provide much more expansive support around these topics.

Oppression is an experience of a person (or group of people) chronically mistreated by a social system or another group, especially from one that typically holds more power or is a predominant group within society. When someone experiences oppression or simply anticipates possible prejudice, the nervous system increases its stress response.[4] Also, research found that oppression in all forms is traumatizing.[5] This is important because, as you've read in this book, reduced stress and processed trauma are critical components for a healthy sexual arousal system.

Also, belief systems (or stereotypes) about oppressed and historically marginalized genders and ethnicities negatively impact general wellness, workplace equity, sexual functioning, and relationships.[6] Sexual stereotypes and experiencing oppression can cause sexual challenges, dissatisfaction, sexual pain, and disappointment disproportionately when compared to non-oppressed groups.[7]

Ableism and neurotypical expectations limit access to care and support for people who have disabilities, complex or chronic Post-Traumatic Stress Disorder, and neurodivergence (Autism, Attention Deficit Disorder, and Attention Deficit Hyperactivity Disorder). Folks with "invisible disabilities" who seem to function in everyday life but struggle internally or at home feel the need to keep on a mask that others in their life expect them to. Dealing with pressures or discrimination based on these experiences creates an impact on daily life as well as intimate and sex lives.

Following are some of the experiences I've heard from clients, friends, and colleagues or read about in research or historically marginalized authored texts.

- Racial stereotypes about a person don't let them experience sex and relationships in the way they want if their desires conflict with the stereotype.

- Women or femmes are expected to be the "caretakers" even though they have the same responsibilities outside of the home or with children as male partners.

- Dealing with micro-aggressions throughout the day.

- Madonna-Whore complex: a heterosexual man has a difficult time experiencing his partner as both erotic or sexually desirable and nurturing or emotionally supportive.

- Being paid less at work than heterosexual, male, or white colleagues for the same level of work and title within the company.

- Healthcare workers don't believe the pain level or severity of medical concerns or conditions due to ethnic or racial stereotypes.

- Experiencing assumptions about relationship status or sexual health status based on stereotypes.

- White, Eurocentric, able-bodied standards of beauty and representation in media and porn.

- Research conducted primarily on white American males informs medical care and treatment for everyone.

- Someone says, "But you look so normal!" when disclosing a disability.

If any of the above or other oppressive, prejudiced, or discriminatory experiences resonate with you, your sexual experiences might be impacted. You can explore this further by asking yourself the following questions:

- When reflecting on experiences of discrimination, how does it affect my perception of personal power?

- How does discrimination make me feel when I think about my body sovereignty or body autonomy?
- How does it impact my energy throughout the day?
- How does it impact how I feel about my partner? Does my partner unknowingly contribute to the discriminatory belief systems or stereotypes I face?
- What are expectations I have for myself and my body that might contribute to the discriminatory belief systems or stereotypes I encounter?

Relationship Challenges Can Shut Down Sexual Arousal and Escalate Avoidance

New research suggests there are two types of "low arousal" for women: *Sexually Dissatisfied* and *Globally Distressed*. The former group is unhappy with their sex life but generally satisfied with their relationship. They often attribute low arousal to external or medical issues. The latter group is dissatisfied with both their relationship and sex life, usually citing their partner or the relationship itself as the cause for low arousal. These attributions show that relationship difficulties can impact sexual satisfaction and arousal for anyone, regardless of gender or orientation.[8] Attachment styles also affect sexual satisfaction. Those with anxious or avoidant attachment styles often feel less satisfied and more disconnected from their partners.[9]

Given this and other research, I wholeheartedly believe difficulties in a partnership can likely cause issues with sexual satisfaction and low arousal regardless of gender, sexual orientation, or relationship dynamic.[10]

As you have learned throughout this book, nervous system regulation is crucial for sexual well-being. Relationship tension, conflict, or poor communication make it harder to relax and access arousal. Partners in conflict often struggle with resolving common issues, such as:

- **Division of Labor:** Imbalances in household responsibilities and emotional labor.

- **Sexual Initiation and Activities:** Prioritizing one partner's pleasure, routine sex, lack of flirting, and one partner always initiating.

- **Communication Issues:** Feeling ignored or misunderstood, cyclical conversations, and differences in what constitutes meaningful conversation.

- **Values:** Conflicts around spending time with friends and family, spirituality, having children, and future plans.

Exploring these topics can be crucial for your sexual well-being if you and your partner don't align on them and you experience constant tension whenever they come up.

In other cases, if you struggle with sex and your partner seems upset, disappointed, or rejected as a result, it will further create pressure and activate or maintain the Sexual Aversion Cycle.

Let's say it's the reverse, and you're feeling disappointed in your sex life due to your partner's difficulty with arousal or sex. Understandably, you would have feelings about your sex life not being what you thought it would be. Many clients in that position express feeling rejected, undesirable, and lonely.

I've had countless conversations with my clients and their partners about how a sexual challenge in one person can cause a strained experience for the partner without the apparent sexual challenge. The key is recognizing that the issue is not the person's fault but a shared challenge, and the partners can work together to find solutions.

Frequently throughout my work with couples, we uncover that both partners ultimately have challenges with sex, even if they initially sought services for only one person.

Case Study: Jackie (she/her) and Rory (he/him)

This couple came in because Jackie had "low arousal," and they both wanted to have more sex. However, Jackie was not as interested in sex lately, and Rory was often feeling rejected when he would attempt to initiate.

After exploring the relationship satisfaction, we learned that there were a lot more emotionally intimate struggles going on, such as Rory's lack of emotional availability, the inequitable division of house labor, and that Rory's attempts to initiate were immediately sexual (for instance, he would grab her butt or breasts to let her know he wanted sex).

As we explored deeper, we uncovered that Rory felt insecure about his body and sexual knowledge. Hence, his efforts in initiating were due to anxiety around his sexual skill set and his performance.

After addressing sharing household chores and creating more time for the couple to have connected conversations, they identified ways to initiate that helped them both "warm up." If we're using the Sexy Time Track as a metaphor, they built longer on-ramps to sexual initiation and activities to reduce anxiety and increase enjoyment for both.

Long-term partnerships often experience a drop in sexual satisfaction after the "honeymoon" phase. According to the well-known couples' therapist, Esther Perel, maintaining a balance between familiarity and novelty is critical to keeping erotic energy alive. Familiarity brings comfort and intimacy, while novelty adds excitement and fantasy. Too much of one can dampen sexual arousal.[11]

For instance, if you have been in a relationship for a long time and have seen your partner on their "less-than-shiny-days" (such as taking care of them when they're sick, or have morning breath, or maybe they've used the restroom with the door open), you have a deep level of intimacy and closeness. However, if you never convey erotic vitality through novel experiences or play, then things can become stale or predictable.

Conversely, suppose you *only* have new partners or mysterious or intense experiences. Building intimacy and connection can be more challenging due to a lack of consistency or sense of security.

I've seen my clients struggle with a "stalled out" sexual relationship with partners because they don't put enough effort into courting, flirting, or dating activities in their long-term relationship the way they first did in the beginning. Not only does this reduce the possibility of staying curious about who your partner is (we're constantly changing and evolving, after all), but it also reduces the opportunities for sexual "priming."

To understand the impact of priming, think about the start of a long-term relationship. The energy was exciting and fresh—you didn't know what it was going to be like to kiss them or see their naked body. So, you probably spent a lot more time fantasizing about this. Your dates with them were a mixture of connection and mystery, so there was more erotic energy. Your thoughts about your partner were about the fun, inspiring future, and sexual potential.

After some time, however, you know what it's like to kiss them. You've seen their body and know what they enjoy sexually. You've talked about where you want the relationship to head. There's much less mystery.

As we've discussed in chapters about the brain, our brains like to create shortcuts. This happens in sex, too. Suppose you know your partner likes that "one thing," and it's reliable to get them aroused or help them arrive at orgasm. In that case, your brain will likely encourage you to go down that well-worn pathway instead of exploring their body, looking for cues to suggest they like what you're doing, or mixing it up with something entirely new. Since you know them so well, you tend to spend less time sexually "priming" yourself. Instead, your thoughts and conversations with them turn to mundane everyday things.

Taking it even further, if the energy between you two is filled with conflict or dealing with relationship struggles, most of the conversations or thoughts around them might be tense—which is the opposite of sexy.

Also, as you spend more and more time together, it can be easy to take for granted that they'll always be there, so there's less effort in flirting, making out, or other sexual play without the expectation of penetration or orgasm. Sexual interactions start to become black-and-white—you start up the engine with a kiss that leads into that thing they like and then the predictable sex acts that usually result in someone (hopefully everyone) reaching orgasm. Although getting to orgasm is an excellent place to be, it can create an energy that sex is goal-oriented and predictable instead of playful, exciting, and pleasure-focused.

There are many ways in which long-term partnerships struggle with sexual and relationship satisfaction. These challenges can reduce arousal potential and increase avoidance. If the above resonates with you, you can use the skills you've developed and Part 4's intimacy and communication tools. Additionally, the Arousal Architecture® in Part 3 will help you uncover new possibilities for increasing sexual priming and reducing relational barriers.

Kinky and Consensually Non-Monogamous Folks Are on to Something

Although a lot of research and sexual self-help books are about heterosexual cisgender couples, I've seen similar challenges as mentioned above with queer, kinky, and consensually non-monogamous (CNM) or polyamorous people.

Despite facing similar challenges, research shows people in CNM relationships have more opportunities for nurturance and eroticism when compared to monogamous relationships.[12] Also, contrary to what many people think, folks who practice BDSM (bondage and discipline, dominance and submission, sadism and masochism) are no more pathological or distressed than other folks and tend to have high sexual and relationship satisfaction when compared to non-BDSM-oriented folks. These (and other) findings indicate that there's something about CNM and kinky practices that increases sexual and relationship satisfaction.

My money is on the fact that those sexual and lifestyle practices require significant investment in personal and relational development so they can engage with sex and relationships in healthy and respectful ways by regularly using communication tools, self-awareness, and regulation techniques.

You might not be into BDSM and might be perfectly satisfied with a monogamous relationship, but that doesn't mean you can't take a page (or two) out of the books of these folks in ways that still align with your values.

Single Life and Dating Can Create Excitement and Anxiety, Simultaneously

Let's say you're "dating yourself" (a.k.a. single). You might be casually dating others, but you're also having struggles with sexual arousal and satisfaction. While some folks love casually dating, it can also be rife with uncertainty, lack of security, confusing situations, and awkward conversations in a partially or fully sexual context. Further, people who wish to be in a relationship but are engaging in casual sex or dating instead might feel unpleasant emotions, thoughts, and beliefs around their experiences because they don't evolve into committed relationships.

Folks with pelvic pain or sexual challenges typically worry about escalating the relationship for fear of having to disclose what feels like a "dirty secret." They might delay sexual initiation or turn down sexual advances by a new partner because they don't know how to broach the topic of their physical or emotional pain with sex. I'll even work with my clients to craft "the sex talk" when they're navigating these issues with new or potential partners. It can help them feel more in control of their emotions, provide a container and structure to know what they plan to say, and reduce anxiety overall.

Regardless of how well conversations or experiences go when dating, they might still contribute to the Sexual Aversion Cycle, which reinforces the importance of using tools to navigate romantic and sexual experiences with self-awareness, compassion, nervous system regulation, and healthy communication.

The Pressures of Life and Pleasure

Beyond external factors, you'll want to look at your internal experiences. For instance, issues related to your personal mental health, life passion or purpose, and hidden psychological processes that you may or may not realize are essential to explore and address for sexual wellness.

If you're dealing with depression, anxiety, grief, trauma, or life transitions that are clinically distressing (like divorce or a job loss), those will take front and center in your life and put sexual arousal on the backburner (or maybe even put it on a plane with a one-way ticket to Neverland). Confronting those challenges with a trusted professional will make it much easier to improve sexual arousal and pleasure.

Another aspect that can zap sexual energy is if you're not living a "meaningful life" (whatever that means, right?). Unfortunately, there's a lot of pressure to "find purpose." While that concept can be another way external forces make us feel "not good enough," there can be delicious energy that translates into sexual vitality when we live our self-defined, passion-filled, or meaningful lives.

In *Think and Grow Rich*, Napoleon Hill explores a concept called "sexual transmutation," where he highlights that men will often do anything for sex. It inspires them to be resourceful, think outside of the box, and overcome barriers that they might not otherwise do unless motivated by obtaining sex.[13] Let's consider this concept in reverse: if you're feeling excited and inspired in your life, you can transmute that energy into sexual energy and creativity. However, if you're not feeling passion in life or experience a lack of meaning, it would make sense that erotic vitality will be hard to access, too.

A lack of purposeful meaning in your life can be a symptom of various issues, so going into depth about what those are and how to address them would take a whole other book. At least knowing that this can contribute to sexual energy is a starting point to explore further on your own or with a trusted professional or friend. Some interventions to improve passion and purpose could include engaging in hobbies, volunteering for an important cause, donating items or money to a local non-profit, or even using exercise as a form of play, such as with acroyoga, partner exercises, or team sports. Ideally, you want to incorporate things that make you feel energetically "sexy." I don't mean erotically, but it's more like you feel badass, excited, and creative. When my clients can connect to these aspects of their lives, I help them bridge that energy from wherever they feel it in their bodies to their genitals. It's impressive to see the results they have with that simple exercise.

In *The Subtle Art of Not Giving a F*ck*, author Mark Manson explains how to invest your time and energy in more passionate ways that reduce burnout. One lesson that stood out to me is aiming to identify meaningful core values that contribute to society, are based in reality, and have an immediate and controllable effect that can help you live a life that feels more energetically aligned with what's important to you. They don't have to be massive goal-oriented values or actions; they can be as simple as "honesty," which hits all values-driven markers mentioned previously.[14]

Alternatively, you might feel mentally stable, healthy, and connected to passion or purpose. You still might not want to have sex. You could be simply tired—too tired for sexual arousal or sex. That's real, especially with our culture's pervasive expectations to be productive. Sex doesn't have to be a priority right now for you, and that's okay!

Recognizing that you might have too much on your plate and want sex to be a priority means you'll want to readjust your priorities when you're ready. Once you are, reflect on the current priorities of your life and what you would like your life to look like six months, a year, or three years from now. Then, work backward to determine what steps you need to take to create your preferred lifestyle, one step at a time. After you've narrowed it down to bite-sized chunks of changes to implement, focus on the next step.

Let's consider a few notable barriers that might also impact your ability to invest energetically in sexual arousal and pleasure.

Guilt-Shame Spiral: Sucking Sexual Energy Right Out of the Room

One of the most common problems I see in sexual challenges is the guilt-shame spiral. We've talked a bit about guilt and shame as it relates to sex. However, suppose your mental processes contain guilt and shame about everyday things. In that case, you'll need to interrupt that spiral to break oppressive internal systems keeping you from a fulfilled life (both in and out of the metaphorical bedroom).

Let's break down guilt and shame because many people get them mixed up or don't even recognize they're experiencing them. A word to my perfectionists—this section will be particularly beneficial for you. As a recovering perfectionist, I needed many profound lessons and constant reminders to stop this process.

Guilt is when you feel responsible or regretful for doing something you believe was an offense, even if that offense is "imagined." It might be when you snap at a colleague, friend, or partner. It could be when you knowingly cut someone off in traffic and pretended you didn't notice. You might also feel guilt when you turn your partner down for sex again. It can come up when you masturbate or indulge in pleasure. Some of those are real (snapping at a human), but others are "imagined," meaning they might not be an offense, but your brain, body, or belief systems tell you it's "wrong." Guilt sounds like "I screwed up."

Shame is when you apply judgment toward yourself about committing an offense, as described above. Shame can be socially helpful and healthy when you identify things about yourself that you dislike because your behaviors don't align with your values. It can motivate you to instigate changes. Healthy shame sounds like, "Ughh, I really don't like that I criticized my partner, again. They've told me how painful it is for them, and acting that way doesn't fit who I want to be."

However, shame can be toxic when it's applied to something out of your control or when you're just beating yourself up over something without using your awareness to take action to improve the situation or how you feel. Toxic shame sounds like, "I'm a terrible person [or partner] because of [this thing]."

Most of my clients realize that the messages they gained from their conservative backgrounds or communities impacted sex without even knowing, for instance, concepts like "indulging in any kind of pleasure can be sinful," "the purpose of a relationship is to procreate," or "thinking of yourself first, instead of your family, is selfish." As we explored in previous chapters, there are still wonderful ways to maintain the values of significant belief systems, such as religious or cultural values, while uprooting ones you believe are holding you back from personal wellness and sexual satisfaction.

Case Study: Amy (she/her)

Amy regularly found herself in a spiral of guilt-shame when she wanted to take a weekly bath because it meant she wasn't available to her family for those thirty minutes. She saw it as selfish and indulgent. She also had difficulty with arousal, pleasure, and orgasm because she would often have sex with her partner in a way that pleased her partner and didn't focus at all on doing what she liked herself. Their sex felt performative for her.

I asked her to take inventory throughout the day when she noticed she felt guilty or had thoughts about herself that triggered shame. Amy realized that most of her thoughts fed the guilt-shame spiral and made her believe she wasn't a good enough partner or mother.

She used the exercise at the end of this chapter to help her reframe her belief about taking care of her own needs. Amy redefined "good enough" to give her more space to make "mistakes," be more present, and recognize that she couldn't "fill from an empty cup."

Amy connected with parts of herself that were more carefree and happier, so she was more engaged with her family and partner. This process, along with the Arousal Architecture®, helped Amy identify and focus on her own sexual needs, allowing her to connect to arousal more quickly, enjoy the experiences more fully, and finally reach orgasm when she wanted to!

In the *Going Deeper* exercise, you'll find an expansion on a familiar process we've already explored at length. Here's a quick guide around guilt and shame and how to reframe them; it's adapted from an Instagram post by therapist Jacquelyn Tenaglia, LMHC (@no.bs.therapist), that captured my attention.[15]

- *Guilt*: I screwed up.
- *Shame*: I'm a screw-up.
- *Blame*: You screwed up.
- *Reframe*: We all screw up—it's a part of life.
- *Accountability*: I screwed up and I will address it.
- *Growth Mindset/Empowerment*: Screw-ups are opportunities to learn, grow, and improve.

Accountability is an integral part of building resilience after making mistakes. Admitting the error without beating yourself up and letting someone else know you're aware of what happened can significantly ease the burden or pain you feel. It's a hard pill to swallow to admit when you might have done something wrong, but regularly practicing healthy accountability is a salve to the deep wound shame causes.

Performative Pleasure: Giving Away the Sexual Energy

Engaging in activities or sex where your focus is providing service, hard work, or pleasure for someone else, and you aren't receiving anything meaningful in return, will ultimately leave you feeling drained or cause burnout. I often see this with clients who are C-suite or high-level executives, therapists, doctors, entrepreneurs, and parents whose children still live at home.

Performative sex can reflect someone's tendencies to self-sacrifice in areas of their life beyond sex also. If you're having sex and not asking for your needs or desires to be incorporated into the play, you might want to look at how you're neglecting yourself in other ways, too.

When it comes to sex, think about how you give and receive pleasure: Are you more focused on the other person's pleasure? Imagine how you touch a partner or perform oral sex on them. Are you doing it in a way that you think they like? Or are you doing it in a way that you also like?

If providing pleasure for others, leaving yourself last or totally out of the picture, resonates with you, start noticing what it would be like to engage with others, partners, and sex in ways that you also enjoy. At work, you can try prioritizing joyful moments throughout the day by moving your body, intentionally relaxing, or enjoying a mindful snack or coffee. With your family or partner, you could ask to do something that helps you decompress, such as a walk in the park or your favorite indulgent movie or show, before prioritizing others' preferences (it's not selfish—it's self-preservation!).

With sex, engage mindfully with your partner and touch them in ways that feel good to you (unless they express they don't like it, then try alternatives). Even if you're performing a sex act that typically feels like "giving," you can still do it in a way you like. For instance, instead of using your mouth or tongue in a way you know your partner enjoys, try doing it in a way your body craves or is interested in. Notice how that changes things for you. It might even heighten your partner's pleasure seeing and feeling the shift in the energy around how you're doing it.

Another aspect of pleasure is to understand the "energy of pleasure." When it comes to folks who have struggled with arousal and sex, the concept of "pleasure" can become energetically loaded with pressure, disappointment, and guilt that they're not experiencing pleasure the way they think they should.

If that's you, let's redefine "pleasure" for now until you feel less emotionally burdened by it; *translation*: until you feel neutral when you think about seeking pleasure—I know, that might seem counterintuitive, but if seeking pleasure causes you to feel mostly unpleasant, you need to rewire that brain pathway to seek neutral first.

Even if you don't have struggles with "pleasure" in this way, you can still benefit from this energetic understanding around it. Instead of seeking "sexual pleasure," aim to connect to "sexual enjoyment." This practice calls upon some of the mindset work in the book's first part. Folks can get so caught up in *expecting* sex to be pleasurable that they often forget to enjoy the experience. Seeking enjoyment in your sexual practices will change your relationship with sex and make it easier to expand your pleasure repertoire.

You might have noticed in earlier chapters that I put "non-sexual" in quotations because *almost* all things and experiences can technically be "sexual." You can wire pathways in your brain and body using the energy of pleasure and somatic practices to create sexual vitality with more options than you realize (more on that in Part 3).

How to Increase Sexual Motivation

Although much of what we've discussed is based on external forces, there are ways you can still influence change. You can seek support to address and process barriers. You can also initiate changes by engaging in behaviors that align with your values and interests. We'll explore how to continue rewriting your sexual narrative with some potent techniques that you'll learn about below.

Motivators Toward Pleasure: Why Do You Want to Have Sex?

Most people are confused when I ask them why they want to have sex, because the answers seem obvious:

- "Because it feels good."
- "I want to feel closer to my partner."
- "It makes my partner happy."

Deeper, below the surface of those responses, is the desire to feel wanted, loved, or cared for, among other reasons.

Now, going beyond those motivations, many people have sex for reasons they wouldn't say out loud. When asked, my clients have admitted theirs behind closed doors, often expressing guilt at their disclosure.

- "It's been a long time since we had sex."
- "I'm afraid my partner will leave or cheat on me if I don't."
- "Sex is a great distraction from other feelings I have."
- "I feel insecure or uncomfortable when friends talk about their sex lives because mine is so difficult or non-existent."
- "I feel so far behind people who are my age."
- "I just want to feel normal."
- "Sex shouldn't feel like an obligation or a chore, but it is."

It can be painful to admit if any of the above resonate with you. Still, my job is to push on your discomfort (lovingly and gently) so we can figure out how to address the barriers keeping you stuck in the Sexual Aversion Cycle.

There's a difference between "wanting it" in your body that serves you versus "wanting it" because you believe you have to. It's not your fault, nor is it likely your partner's. You learned about your needs in a sex-negative system based on expectation or pressure and possibly misaligned with values that feel good for you.

There are two different kinds of motivations for having sex.

1. *Expectations or Pressure*: These are societal expectations ("To be a good partner, I should be available sexually," "I'm [a certain age] so I should have had sex by now," or "My partner will leave me if we don't have more sex").

2. *Alignment and Enjoyment*: These healthy reasons best support your needs and align with your values and interests.

Making this distinction for yourself will help you identify when you want it for *you* versus when you're doing it for another reason that might deplete your resources instead of nourishing them. Pinpointing your motivations can reveal issues that need further intervention. You'll also uncover better solutions to increasing arousal and pleasure.

So, think beyond pleasure or connection—ask yourself why you *actually* have sex. You might feel great about the answers. That's fantastic! Use those to optimize your experiences.

Regardless of what you learn about yourself, if you were having the kind of sex you ultimately crave, ask yourself these questions:

- What would it look like?
- Where would you have sex?
- How would you be touched? How would you use touch?
- Who would be with you (if anyone)?
- What would it mean to you?

Of those, determining how you want to feel during and about sex is the most impactful. Let's focus on those now.

Below are some starting points. See if any of these resonate for you or if others come to mind:

- Connected
- Powerful
- Relaxed
- Special
- "Competent"
- Safe, secure in the relationship
- Valued or enjoyed
- Unique connection
- Relationship maintenance

Understanding how you want to feel can help you connect further to why you have sex. You can rewrite a more authentic sexual narrative when inspired by motivations anchored in meaningful values. This is the case whether you enjoy casual sex or polycules or marriage. Someone who enjoys casual sex can be motivated by independence, flexibility, or adventure. There's no wrong answer, only what's right for you. Ideally, you'll reframe your belief system into something that feels less like an obligation or chore and more like an activity that reflects your values, erotic energy, and sexual identity.

After identifying *why* you have sex, the next step is to align your thoughts and behaviors around having sex that fits how you want to feel. Okay, sure, but how do you do that? The short answer: Assess the sexual thoughts and behaviors you're engaging in and determine if they align with your meaningful purpose for having sex. If not, shifts are needed.

Consider someone who has sex because they want to feel regularly desired. They could do any of the following items:

- Decide to be a unicorn for couples.
- Listen to audio erotica where the sexy stranger or lover desires the main character.
- Learn about goddess-worshiping kinks and seek out devotee partners.
- Ask their partner to engage in more flirting and courting behaviors.
- Before direct genital stimulation, touch other areas of their body.
- Ask their partner for comments about how much they want them.

If it feels uncomfortable or challenging to try these in "high-pressure situations," you could first identify ways to do this in low-pressure situations, such as in your solo sexual play or other activities that feel more accessible to start with. Then, using the skills we've explored in the book, pair nervous system regulation to the activity so that it feels more neutral. Then, lean into the ways it feels at least neutral. With time and practice, it can increase confidence and pleasure.

It's also important to note that sometimes, we all have sex for "relationship maintenance." There's nothing wrong with engaging in sexual play because "it's been a while" or as a form of stress relief. The underlying motivators can still align with deeper meaning, such as having sex for health and wellness or keeping the sexual energy alive in your relationship instead of neglecting it because you're too tired. The main distinction is about how it makes you feel and how balanced your intentions are when engaging in sexual play. As long as you genuinely feel good about how and why you have sex, that's what matters.

Rewriting Your Sexual Narrative: Cognitive and Somatic Reframe

Now, we'll weave everything together in a cohesive system for understanding how to rewrite your sexual narrative. You'll have a step-by-step system to use as you learn more about yourself with the Arousal Architecture® in the next part. As you explore your unique arousal design, you might experience tension around your desires and sexual interests. Now, you'll have a tool to navigate them with confidence.

As I mentioned before, I'm not the biggest fan of only using cognitive behavioral therapy (CBT) for sexual or mental health issues. It can be a good starting point, but it's missing the critical element of incorporating your body into your practice.

CBT interventions suggest you challenge thoughts with logical questioning (such as the Alternative Possibilities we explored earlier) to change your reactions to events. As you now know, accessing logic is hard to do when your nervous system is in a threat or trauma response. The logical part of your mind is "offline." To bring it back online, you need to regulate the nervous system (informing the system that it's safe). Then, once it knows it's safe, the logic and language centers can come back online, and at that point, it's easier to access more helpful thoughts.

Even though your brain can consider Alternative Possibilities, how do you believe them in your body? Most of the people I work with express frustration because they know they can tell themselves their partner is "safe," or that they want to be aroused, or want to have sex, but if their bodies don't believe it, what good are words or thoughts going to do? It's like the notion of "thoughts and prayers" in response to school shootings instead of implementing better gun accessibility laws and effective mental health for everyone.

So, using science, somatic methods, and everything you've learned so far, the following is a process for rewriting your sexual narrative, thought by thought or belief by belief. It integrates components of the previous exercises in one cohesive step-by-step system using the NeuroSomaticSex Method™ for Therapy and Coaching. If you use nothing else in this book, I hope you walk away with this at least!

A common CBT technique is cognitive restructuring, which, at its most basic understanding, suggests selecting a thought and feelings associated with it. Then, identify other thoughts that might result in a different experience or behavior (the final step). I've put the CBT steps in the darker boxes in Figure 7.1.

However, with the somatic processes added in (the lighter boxes), you'll find a much more effective framework for rewriting your sexual narrative.

Here's how to use it.

An *Automatic Thought* pops up about a situation. You can't prevent these from occurring. They just happen and are formed out of your past experiences and beliefs. With time and by rewriting your sexual narrative, you'll transform the kind of automatic thoughts that occur.

Next, you notice the *Emotions* that arise. As you've learned, your nervous system responds to your interpretation of situations and creates *Body Sensations*. Unpleasant reactions might indicate your body detects a threat. Most people remain in their heads at this point, trying to figure out how to solve the problem or are spiraling in an emotional cognitive process.

Your aim in this new process is to stay in the body in a way that helps you feel more in control and facilitate change. Do that by engaging in a *Regulating Intervention* (e.g., mindfulness, somatic practice, or other resource that works for you) until you notice mostly neutral sensations.

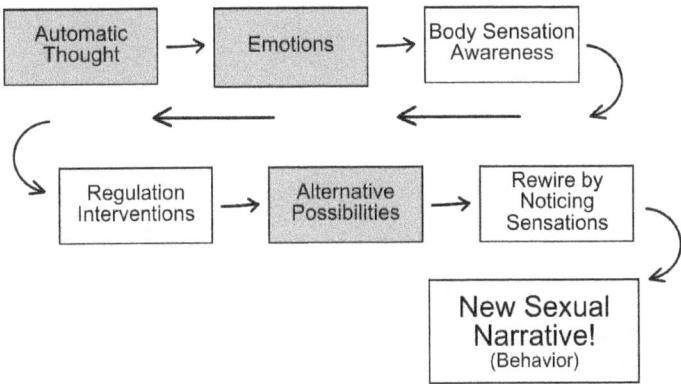

FIGURE 7.1 *Cognitive and Somatic Reframe exercise.*

That will make it much easier to access the Alternative Possibilities because you've brought the logic center in your brain back online to access higher-level parts of your brain instead of the areas governed by survival. You can also assess the situation more clearly when emotions don't hijack you. Now, put on your compassionate scientist hat and explore other meanings, beliefs, or feelings you'd prefer to have that align with your desired values.

The next step is where the magic happens. It's impractical to expect yourself to believe that the new Alternative Possibilities can suddenly become a reality. Instead, you will *Rewire by Noticing Sensations* which "imprints" the new possibility (or belief) into your nervous system.

Do you remember when you learned to seek out pleasant sensations related to Alternative Possibilities or desired beliefs? Do something similar here as well. Focus on sensations in your body that respond pleasantly to this new possibility being accurate, even if that's the tiniest part of your body that says, "Yeah! That's what I believe!" Focus on the sensations in that part of your body, spending at least thirty seconds noticing them and any other neutral or pleasant ones connected to that belief.

By doing this, you're rewiring your brain pathways by creating new nervous system responses to an Automatic Thought that was previously associated with unpleasant associations.

That's the NeuroSomaticSex magic of paving a new pathway in *rewriting your new sexual narrative*!

Figure 7.2 gives an example of how one of my clients used this process.

Although a seemingly simple process, it's not "easy" to do. You won't see change immediately just because you tried this a few times. It takes dedication and repetition. Sometimes, you need more support than just doing it on your own, but if you start with Automatic Thoughts or beliefs that feel "small," you can work up to larger ones.

Being able to identify the motivators for having sex and using your nervous system regulation techniques and new found body sensations to help you pave

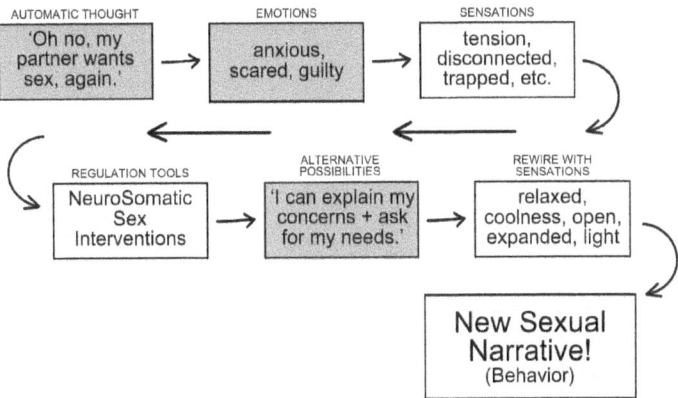

FIGURE 7.2 *An example of using the Cognitive and Somatic Reframe exercise.*

new pathways, you'll be able to harness the energetic experience of arousal, pleasure, and sexual satisfaction into a new way of relating to and expressing your sexual narrative!

Pleasure Gems

- Avoiding sex can be about more than just the act itself. It can include external forces that you may not have control of. You can control how you respond to them, which creates empowerment and confidence.
- Relationship satisfaction influences sexual arousal, so it's crucial to address issues or tension around dating and being intimate in proactive ways.
- Lack of meaning in your life or other mental health challenges can reduce resources for sexual arousal and satisfaction. Connect with alignment and passion as best as possible or seek support to implement change.
- The guilt-shame spiral and performative pleasure are sneaky culprits suppressing more fulfilling sexual experiences. Acknowledging they occur is the first step to overcoming them.

- You can increase sexual arousal and satisfaction by looking at the deeper motivations you have for sex.
- Rewrite your sexual narrative using the Cognitive and Somatic Reframe tool.

Exercises

Quick Wins!

Create Opportunities for Connection or Intimacy

I'm sure you've heard of "scheduling sex." Don't do that—instead, schedule opportunities for connection or intimacy. Remove the pressure on expecting sex. Spend time doing things that help you build up to the *possibility* of sexual play. Then, it will be so much easier to want to engage in sex when the moment arises. Or not. You don't have to if you're not feeling it.

That's the beauty of this exercise—if you don't have a certain kind of "sex," you didn't miss out. You had the kind of experience you intended to have (connection or intimacy).

If you still feel pressure knowing sex is still on the table, remove it from the menu of possibilities. Decide this in advance if you're doing the exercise solo, or talk about it in advance with your partner so you're on the same page. It doesn't have to be a forever decision; try it out for a few weeks and see what that does to your or your partner's experience.

Connect Passionate Energy to Your Genitals

With this exercise, use an experience you are already familiar with and help it fuel your sexual energy.

1. To start, think about something that elicits passion, creativity, or exciting "non-sexual" feelings. Notice what happens in your

body—where do you feel it? What sensations do you notice? Specifically, notice the passionate or pleasurable sensations in your body. Maybe even place a hand on that part of your body. Spend at least thirty seconds doing this.

2. Now, place one hand on your genitals in whatever way you like: over clothes, underwear, or with skin-to-skin contact.

3. Next, imagine creating a bridge connecting your genitals to the "non-sexual" place in your body where you feel the creative, passionate, or exciting energy.

4. Finally, imagine "sending" those sensations across the bridge, noticing what it feels like to experience the same kind of sensations in your genitals.

Even if you don't know if you're "doing it right," the imagined process of "pretending" to notice the sensations or feelings can impact you. Your brain still wires pathways, so give it a shot!

It may take some consistent repetitions to do this. The compound effect is your friend in this practice—the more times you practice, the easier it will be to see the payoff in the long run.

Like your practices earlier in this book, you could commit to trying this daily or at least a few times a week for about two to five minutes.

Going Deeper

Identify Your Off-Ramps

Consider all we've talked about regarding cognitive processes, thoughts, beliefs, body experiences, and energetic influences. Then reflect on what gets in your way of the following:

- Thinking about sex?
- Engaging in sex?

- Being present in sex?
- Feeling aroused?
- Reaching orgasm?

Don't forget to include influences that don't even seem connected to sex (e.g., a partner won't take out the trash as they promised, racism, or guilt about making a mistake at work). You'll have more guidance in Part 3 to get even more specific, so this is a starting point.

Find and Embrace Your On-Ramps

Imagine, eight weeks from now, you've finished the book, you've implemented the lessons and interventions you've learned, and you're having the kind of sex you want.

Paint a picture in your head about what that looks like. What's it like in the morning when you wake up? How are you feeling about yourself? Or about a partner or potential partner? How do you feel as you think about going about your morning routine, knowing you're excited about your sex life? How do you act differently?

Notice the sensations in your body as you think about this.

Use your experience to identify and start a list of your motivators for sex. If it's helpful, refer to the section on motivators to stimulate ideas. These will help you craft more specifics in the following chapters.

Cognitive and Somatic Reframe to Rewrite Your Sexual Narrative

Use the Cognitive and Somatic Reframe in the previous section to confront automatic thoughts that arise when you think about sex or experience unpleasant sensations or emotions, anytime and every time you can. This will rewire your brain pathways. The more you do it, the quicker you'll see that compounding effort.

PART 3

THE AROUSAL ARCHITECTURE®

ar·chi·tec·ture, *noun*: the complex or carefully designed structure of something

Everything you've learned in this book was designed to bring you to this moment.

You now have a foundation for understanding how your "sexual self" came to be. You're armed with neuroscience and research to create sexual wellness. The interventions you've learned will help you navigate difficulties in rewriting your sexual narrative. Knowing yourself and how to deal with metaphorical hiccups in sex will pave the way for increasing sexual satisfaction, no matter if you already have good enough sex and want to optimize it or if you've struggled with sexual issues like anxiety, pain, or disappointment.

Now, you'll use your new skills and lessons to integrate the Arousal Architecture® into your sexual repertoire for authentic arousal, deeper connection, and epic sex.

Sexual satisfaction is more than just a luxury; research has found that it's also necessary for overall wellness. Low sexual satisfaction is linked to health issues, poor quality of life, and even memory decline later in life.[1] As you read in previous chapters, sexual satisfaction is not only based on explicitly sexual behaviors but also on intimacy-based motivations and emotional outcomes of engaging in sex.

We've all been told what "should" happen to our bodies for sexual arousal and pleasure. However, almost everything you've learned about sexual arousal growing up is probably wrong. Your arousal system is much more sophisticated than what our sex-negative society gives you credit for because it's rooted in oppressive systems like heteronormativity and patriarchy.[2] Sexual "standards" need to be reevaluated.

> But that's just the way it is!
> I can't get my partner to change.
> I don't even know where to start—the usual sexual things don't turn me on, so I guess there's no hope.
> I've never really felt connected to my sexual arousal; I don't know what works for me.

These are typical concerns I've heard as a therapist and coach when my clients have worked through their pain or "threat response" to sex. They had been in so much pain or had no concept of their sexual self because their "sexual self" had been wholly oppressed since childhood. The idea of creating possibilities for more appealing sexual situations felt foreign. Most clients previously tried sex or intimacy workshops or online programs to help them "reignite the passion" or "claim the sexual power within." Although those offerings are probably great for a lot of people, most of my clients needed a bridge to get from where they were (recovering from a threat or trauma response to sex and arousal) to a place where they could incorporate those models into their sexual narrative without feeling self-conscious about their current sexual state.

After years of hearing the same needs, I created Arousal Architecture®. It has evolved for over a decade based on thousands of hours of clinical interviews and practical applications. This revolutionary model transformed my clients' lives because it met them where they were regardless of how much sex they had, what they desired, or who they were having sex with (or not!).

My clients finally felt hopeful when we normalized that there isn't a "norm" for sexual arousal. Further, they loved learning how to tap into resources in areas of their lives (that didn't seem related to their sex lives) to transform their sexual satisfaction.

Although initially developed for folks who have had challenges with sexual arousal, anxiety, and pain, the Arousal Architecture® can also help anyone who wants to uncover new and unique ways to become aroused. Furthermore, it builds resilience and mental health for overall wellness.

If you're familiar with *The 5 Love Languages*®, it's like that but for your arousal system.[3] The Arousal Architecture® gives you a much more flexible and expansive understanding of what you need for easier access to optimizing your sexual arousal system. It motivates you to seek general pleasure (or joy) in all areas of life. When you can connect to pleasure with less pressure or expectation, you build confidence and a skill set by knowing what it's like to feel joy and pleasure in little (but profound) ways.

8

Your Unique Arousal System

The Arousal Architecture® is your unique design for sexual, sensual, intimate, and erotic pleasure potential. It's informed by science and the mind-body connection. Your results from taking the Arousal Architecture® assessment will help you conceptualize your unique sexual arousal system beyond sexual preferences. The results honor genetic and hereditary factors, upbringing, desired values, and experiences you've had throughout life. With the Arousal Architecture®, you'll have a tangible way to categorize your on-ramps and off-ramps so you can optimize your arousal potential with a systematic process. It might not sound sexy, but just wait until you see the results!

In this chapter, we'll define some key terms to help you expand your sexual arousal toolbox. You'll learn how the Arousal Architecture® will help you unlock sexual satisfaction without pressure as a non-judgmental, inclusive, and supportive model. You'll learn to look at your arousal potential from a lens of compassion and curiosity instead of tension or self-criticism.

Key Definitions for Understanding the Power of the Arousal Architecture®

Why Is It an *Architecture*?

In the Arousal Architecture® model, "architecture" refers to the sophisticated construction of your sexual arousal. It acknowledges you are a holistic being, incorporating your brain (e.g., belief systems, values), body (e.g., nervous system, threat responses, sense of safety), and energy (e.g., meaning, culture, society).

I like using metaphors when explaining seemingly abstract concepts such as sexual arousal. You can conceptualize your arousal system and sense of your sexual self as a multi-story building. A building needs a solid foundation before it can serve a purpose. I hope you gained a supportive foundation through the lessons you learned in the book's first two parts.

While a building is under construction, proper scaffolding is needed to build it quickly and safely. The Arousal Architecture® is the scaffolding to construct your sexual self.

Notable Phrases in the Arousal Architecture® Model

You've encountered some of these terms before, and we'll refer to them as we continue:

- *Arousal potential*: Your ability to access sexual arousal easily. It is related to sexual arousal and how much of it you can acquire with this model.

- *Pleasure potential*: Your ability to access pleasure easily. This includes joy, enjoyment, or overall pleasurable sensations, not just sexual pleasure.

- *Arousal language*: Refers to your arousal needs, desires, or aspects of life that make arousal or pleasure easier to access. Similar to Love Languages®, but more dimensional.

- *Authentic arousal (and pleasure)*: These are the genuine arousal and pleasure-based needs and desires you have based entirely on who you are and what you want. They are part of your holistic identity, including your sexual identity. Your authentic arousal or pleasure is not informed by toxic expectations, gender roles, societal or cultural "norms," stereotypes, or anything else that feels oppressive to you. These aspects of your identity might look different than your partner's and are just as valid and celebrated!
- *Sexual self*: A part of your overall identity that connects to your sexuality and sexual wellness. Your sexual self isn't limited to sexual situations; you can utilize skills from the Arousal Architecture® to evolve and expand your sexual self and sex life in appropriate and accessible ways. Also, it includes your arousal and pleasure potentials, arousal language, and authentic arousal and pleasure.

Now that you understand these concepts, let's dive into what the Arousal Architecture® truly is.

About the Arousal Architecture® Assessment and Your Results

The Arousal Architecture® assessment is a questionnaire structured to reveal your unique sexual arousal design by evaluating five specific dimensions. Here's what you need to know to take the assessment and understand your results:

Taking the Assessment

During the assessment, you will answer a series of questions to help you determine your Arousal Architecture®. At the time of writing this book, it's fifty questions and takes about ten to fifteen minutes. However, we're working on evolving it and creating an even more robust process, so you might have a slightly different option if you choose to access the assessment online.

You can take the assessment and obtain your results in two different ways:

1. Use the written assessment questions at the end of this chapter. There, you'll find instructions on answering questions and scoring your results.

2. Go to www.arousalarchitecture.com and answer the questions online (we don't store your responses to keep the assessment confidential). You'll get your results immediately, and the total scores also will be emailed to you. Plus, if you take it online, you will get a free e-book with an overview of the content and a downloadable workbook as you continue through the rest of this book. You'll also get updates about more innovative ways to use your Arousal Architecture® results, along with interventions I love gifting to my community.

Understanding Your Arousal Architecture® Results

Your results will consist of five different numbers, each ranging from 0 to 10, representing your total in the following dimensions:

- Sexual Stimulation
- Embodied Experience
- Mental Headspace
- Energetic Connection
- Erotic Exploration

Your total reflects how *influential* each dimension is in creating arousal for you. There isn't a "better" or "worse" total. If you get a low number, it means that dimension is less critical for you to access arousal. A high number means it's something that helps construct your arousal language.

Learning About the Arousal Architecture® Dimensions

In the following five chapters, you'll learn the details about each dimension. We'll dive deep into what they mean, how to use them to improve your arousal and pleasure potentials, and how to change the influence of the dimension if that's what you want.

However, if you're in a hurry to get a general overview of each dimension and want to implement techniques as soon as possible, the e-book and workbook with the online assessment will be the fast lane for you.

Importance of Each Dimension

Some dimensions may significantly influence your arousal, while others might have a lesser impact. Your totals will help identify which areas are most relevant to you and which you might consider adjusting.

Just because you score high in a dimension, it does not mean that it positively influences your sexual self. You might score high in a dimension like Mental Headspace because you're often in your head and have difficulty being fully present. In that case, you could use interventions to reduce cognitive spirals or thought patterns and increase nervous system regulation through somatic practices.

Your number within a dimension is just data—there's no right or wrong answer to the questions and no goal to reach 0 or 10 in any dimension. Don't judge or critically compare your levels between dimensions or against others who take the Arousal Architecture®. The results help you learn about yourself, what turns you on, and possibilities for accessing enhanced arousal.

If you are concerned about your dimension total—if you want any total to be higher or lower—you can adjust them using interventions my clients have found helpful. I'll provide some in each chapter.

As discussed in the metaphor, the Arousal Architecture® is like scaffolding. Think of the dimensions as planks or paths in the scaffolding, which help you access tools for improving your arousal and pleasure.

There's nothing wrong with what you want or what you need to feel good in your body and about sex. You'll learn that each dimension has its benefits and support systems to enhance your experience, no matter what your total number is in any of them.

Most importantly, by using the Arousal Architecture®, you will learn that your sexual system isn't broken.

Practical Examples of Using the Arousal Architecture®

Once you have your results and understand each dimension, you can use this information in various ways. You'll have an innovative understanding of your sexual self, which will help you better understand your body and arousal system.

Harmful belief systems, adverse experiences, or other difficulties might make it difficult for someone to express their sexual self the way they desire. By understanding and applying the insights from your assessment, you can better navigate your sexual arousal and enhance your intimate experiences.

You'll also learn to identify items (such as thoughts, behaviors, or experiences) that will help increase your arousal potential and provide concrete requests to share with a partner so they can contribute to building sexual arousal with you.

Furthermore, knowing a partner's needs and how their body might work similarly or differently to yours can significantly enhance your relationship. With this knowledge and the tools provided in Part 4, you can have more effective and fulfilling conversations with your partner(s).

Case Study: Jessi (she/her) and Ben (he/him)

Let's look at an Arousal Architecture® design of a former client who struggled with low arousal and painful sex (dyspareunia) due to medical conditions (vestibulodynia and vaginismus). Jessi first started working with me individually for pelvic pain treatment.

Figure 8.1 shows Jessi's results (labeled Partner A). Her Arousal Architecture® design reflects low numbers with Sexual Stimulation and Erotic Exploration, which means that those dimensions are less influential in her arousal system at this point (it could change over time, but more on that later). She has higher numbers for Embodied Experience, Mental Headspace, and Energetic Connection, which means that those dimensions are more influential in her joy, pleasure, and sexual arousal.

Once Jessi completed our "Overcoming Painful Sex Program," she and her partner, Ben, engaged in our "Couple's Pleasure Program."

Physically painful sex impacts more than a person's body and sexual arousal. It also alters someone's interest in intimacy, relationship satisfaction, and the partner's relationship to sex. Jessi and Ben's situation was no different. They needed to work on interrupting the relationship's Sexual Aversion Cycle now that the pain in Jessi's body had largely resolved.

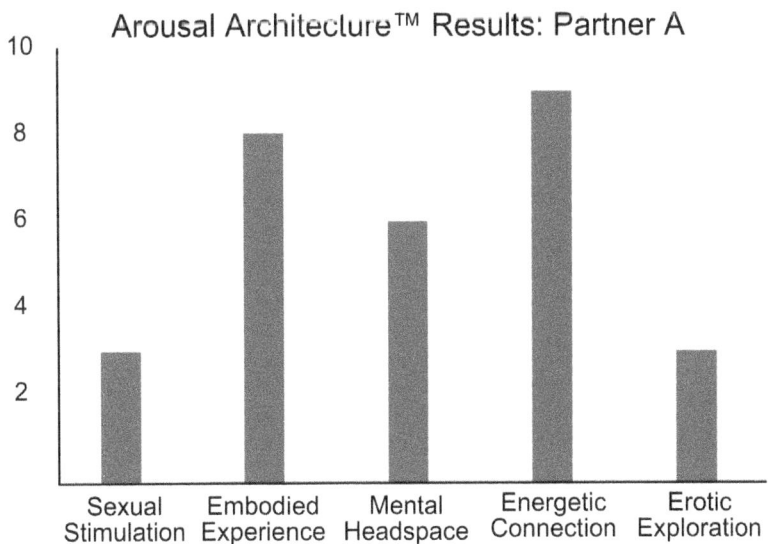

FIGURE 8.1 *The Arousal Architecture® results for Partner A.*

Ben wanted spontaneous, playful, and creative sexual experiences at least three times per week. On the other hand, Jessi was often tired during the week, focused on the kids during the weekends, and desired to feel more emotionally and mentally connected with Ben.

When not working, they typically spent their time in front of screens or dealing with the house and kids, and there was little time left for the light-hearted intimacy they had when they started dating. This couple thought they had lost the "spark" since they had been together for so long and had dealt with so much pain and discomfort with sex. These were the off-ramps for the couple. The emotions they felt around their sex lives revealed a Sexual Aversion Cycle that occurred for years before the painful sex even began. Jessi and Ben both felt resentment, guilt, and disappointment about what their sex life devolved to.

In Figure 8.2, you'll see Ben's Arousal Architecture® results (labeled Partner B) compared with Jessi's, which I used to develop interventions for them.

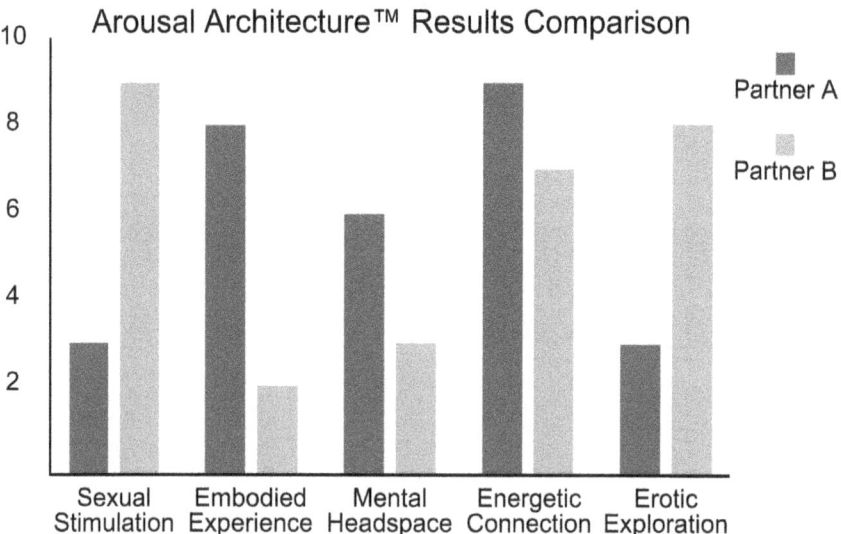

FIGURE 8.2 *The Arousal Architecture® results comparison between Partners A and B.*

Using the Arousal Architecture® results and exercises, they realized it wasn't about one person being right or wrong in their desires or needs. Instead, they realized they needed to better understand each other's arousal language. The key was to move away from blame, shame, doubt, and problem-focused mindsets and toward a mutual understanding and respect for their unique needs for sexual arousal and pleasure.

You can have these shifts, too!

Applying the Model to Expand Your Arousal and Pleasure Potential

To understand the substance of your personalized results and how to use the Arousal Architecture® dimensions in your life, refer to the assessment questions and how you answered them. I'll guide you in ways similar to what we do in our programs. You'll uncover the significance of your answers and how to leverage that information to enhance your arousal or pleasure potential. In Chapter 14, I'll provide a detailed example to further illustrate the real-world application of the Arousal Architecture®.

To do this for yourself, you'll see that each of the following five chapters has the same structure for the *Going Deeper* exercises, explained below. There are also prompts to help you learn more about or explore each specific dimension.

Going Deeper Exercise Instructions

1. Reflect on the questions you had passionate responses to. It can be any question; it doesn't have to be ones you responded "Mostly True" to because even a "Mostly False" can provide valuable insight into your arousal language.

For example, in the Mental Headspace dimension, maybe you responded, "Heck yeah!" to the question, "Sexy music helps me stay present, and if good jams are on, I can consider getting in the mood." Then that's one of the questions you'll dive deeper into.

2. Get detailed about your answers to those questions. Imagine looking at your response with a fine-toothed comb, wanting to know everything about it.

Because what does "sexy music" actually mean? It's probably different for me than you, and for other reasons as well. Since the goal of the Arousal Architecture® is to help you more deeply understand the architecture of your sexual self, you need to get detailed to create awareness and bring more meaning to the surface. You can go as deep as you want, but the more you understand *what* you enjoy and *why*, the better your arousal system and sex life will be.

For instance, ask yourself what kind of music can get you in the mood? What kind of music *doesn't* do it for you? Does it need to be instrumentals only, or do you like lovely soft vocals? Do you like heavy bass or light romantic love songs? Get explicit about the details.

3. Then, go a little further by interviewing yourself using a "5W and H" journalism technique by asking who, what, when, where, why, and how as it relates to your "Mostly True" or "Mostly False" responses.

Think back to the motivators you identified in the previous chapter. How do you want to feel regarding the scenario the question asks about? Are there certain situations when you might want something else in a different rendition of that situation?

To explain this a little further, I'm going to share a little about my own experience: I have Attention Deficit Hyperactivity Disorder, and music with prominent lyrics in the song is too distracting when I'm trying to stay in my body. Also, when some songs have associated memories, it often triggers an off-ramp because I start thinking about those memories instead of the potential pleasure in my body.

So, if I wanted to set the ambiance for a satisfying sexual experience, I would choose an instrumental mix that I don't listen to regularly. It would be sensual and have good bass or percussions at a decibel level that most would describe as "background" noise. However, in certain circumstances, like when I want to feel powerful and have more primal experiences, I would put on my loud "Vampire Party/Dark Clubbing" mix.

The idea is to understand *why* you answered the way you did, along with any detail that can help you expand your understanding of your arousal needs and sexual self.

As you discover the meaning of your responses and how they influence your sexual self and your arousal language, you can unlock experiences that will increase joy, arousal, and pleasure in ways you might not have realized were available to you.

The Differences and Power of the Arousal Architecture® Model

Many folks have linked the well-known 5 Love Languages® or Erotic Blueprint® models to the Arousal Architecture® model, which I always find incredibly flattering since they were instrumental in my inspiration and creation process. The connection to these models makes sense pragmatically because they all conceptualize arousal and sexual pleasure in a structured way, with the understanding that a variety of experiences map out our intimacy and arousal systems and how we relate to partners.

However, unlike those and other models, the Arousal Architecture® is not just about love, intimacy, or sex. It's about personal transformation. It's about finding parts of yourself that can increase joy and set the stage for arousal in a way that's uniquely yours. Some other notable differences can help you understand how the Arousal Architecture® can support an even more profound transformation, which I'll discuss later.

#1 A Dynamic Model

The Arousal Architecture® doesn't provide one or two fixed profiles. Instead, it's a more flexible way to look at your desires and sexuality. Our sexual arousal response systems might change over time, between partners, or depending on where you're at in your life. Since our sexuality flows and transforms, this model provides multiple paths to navigate those shifts to support you. The other models can offer this as well; you just retake the quiz and might have a new profile based on your potentially new answers. However, the Arousal Architecture® model already incorporates into your results that you're a dynamic person from week to week, situation to situation, and so on. Although, with significant life changes, retaking the Arousal Architecture® can provide an updated design if you feel it's necessary.

Additionally, the dimensions can overlap with each other, recognizing that we're not limited to a singular personification of your assessment results. Rather, it honors the many parts of who you are and what works for you in multiple ways. Figure 8.3 reflects the concept of the Arousal Architecture® more accurately than graphs since it captures its dynamic characteristics better.

The image at the top of Figure 8.3 reflects all the Arousal Architecture® dimensions, and the one at the bottom demonstrates what the dimension circles would look like for Jessi from the earlier case study.

Notice how something that arouses you or adds to your pleasure or joy can be in multiple dimensions. Also, the same thing that arouses you can be in a different dimension for someone else. Or they can be turned on by it for a different reason than you are.

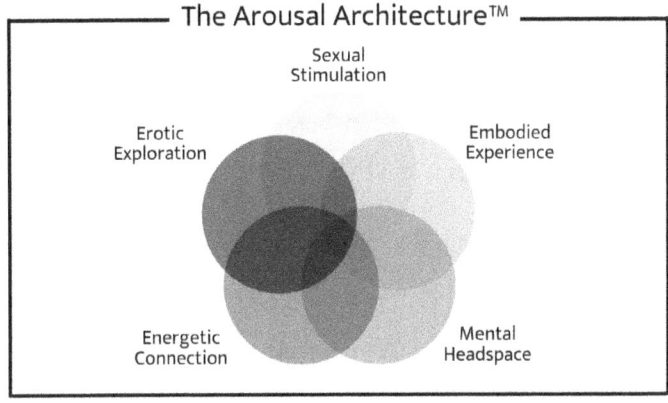

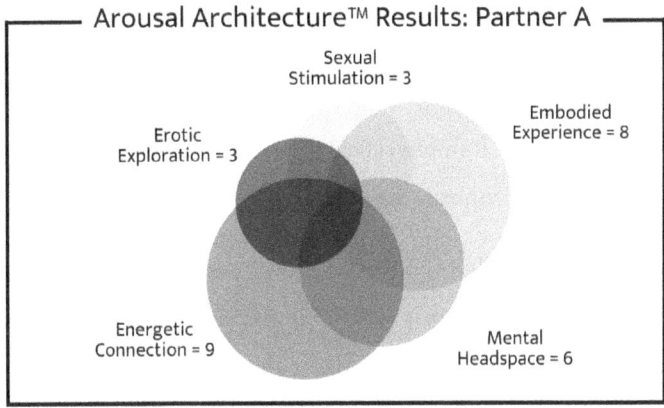

FIGURE 8.3 *The Arousal Architecture® circles and example results where each dimension's circle size is adjusted for the level of importance based on the assessment results.*

It's a complex model, I know. But don't worry; I promise there won't be a pop quiz later.

The bottom line is to know that this is a fluid model to adapt to our fluctuations around pleasure, arousal, and sex. The central concept to hold on to is knowing *why* you enjoy or get turned on by something. This understanding can help you access new ideas and ways to increase your arousal that you might not have realized.

At this point, it might all seem abstract, so here's an example to make it more tangible.

Case Study: Kate (she/her)

Kate sometimes enjoys being hugged or held from behind by a sexual or romantic partner. This behavior can belong to one or more dimensions, depending on why Kate likes it and the meaning she assigns it.

- *Sexual Stimulation*: Experiencing her partner's body pressed against hers feels explicitly sexual, especially when they are naked.
- *Embodied Experience*: It makes her feel safe and grounded.
- *Mental Headspace*: She interprets that this means she is petite and taken care of.
- *Energetic Connection:* She feels close and connected to her partner.
- *Erotic Exploration*: It might reflect a power dynamic that she enjoys (her partner is in control over her, consensually).

Before using the Arousal Architecture®, Kate was confused about why this action felt arousing and exciting when one partner did it but uncomfortable when another tried. Kate realized that she enjoyed the feeling of closeness and submission with her female partner. However, trying it with her male partner felt too similar to an unpleasant experience with a different male partner. By using interventions and understanding from the Arousal Architecture®, Kate found options with her male partner that helped her feel petite, connected, and submissive in a power dynamic that didn't activate a threat response.

Exploring the impact and meanings of the dimensions helped Kate remove shame and guilt from her sexual response with male partners. It enabled her to unlock more possibilities and increase options for on-ramps.

#2 The Arousal Architecture® Disrupts the Sexual Aversion Cycle and Threat Response

Folks who are in constant tension with their partner around sex and intimacy or have had one too many failed relationships eventually find themselves in a Sexual Aversion Cycle.

In many situations within a relationship, one partner can access arousal more quickly than the other. Those folks can be turned on by what society says is "typical" or "normal" to be aroused by: they can see their partner naked or get excited about simply making out, or maybe they can watch porn and be aroused in moments. With a spontaneous desire, they can easily anticipate pleasure from those possibilities.

Meanwhile, their partner feels pressured to be aroused at the same level or speed. When that doesn't happen in the "expected way," guilt and dissatisfaction appear in the bedroom, uninvited.

Cue the Sexual Aversion Cycle.

So, which partner do you think is the "healthiest" sexually? Trick question! It doesn't mean that one partner is healthier than the other. Far from it, in fact.

Neither partner is "wrong," "broken," or "demanding" by needing more time or different kinds of stimulation to become aroused—it just means that they both need to learn the many other ways that they can turn each other on and start to speak each other's arousal language better. That's where the Sexual Pleasure Paradigm Shift from Chapter 6 can help.

Instead of staying stuck in the Sexual Aversion Cycle, you can bring the process to the surface, acknowledge what you notice about yourself, and use the interventions in this book with the Arousal Architecture® to interrupt the pattern.

My clients find that when they envision their arousal potential from this new paradigm and embrace the newly revealed arousal needs, their relationships and sexual satisfaction improve!

#3 Arousal Architecture® Helps with Responsive Desire

Another essential aspect of the Arousal Architecture® is understanding that sometimes some folks need a longer on-ramp for accessing sexual arousal than others. They might also prefer to experience more intimacy-based needs in their sexual experience than only the physical act of sex. Again, this is not because of a broken arousal system. Cultural expectations and lessons around sexual arousal have prioritized people who have easy access to their arousal, much like how our society prioritizes penis pleasure and penis-in-vagina sex.

Identifying the expansive aspects of joy, pleasure, and sexual arousal helps someone who has responsive desire, especially if their arousal language reflects that they seek emotional intimacy from sexual play or prefer more time connecting before shifting to explicitly sexual interactions.

The Arousal Architecture® isn't only an answer for people with responsive desire; it can also enhance the sex lives of folks with spontaneous desire and everyone in between. It simply provides an easier way to conceptualize and verbalize everyone's unique and expansive needs.

#4 It Removes the Pressure from Focusing on Sexual Pleasure

As we've explored in Part 2, pressure is a total arousal killer. The Arousal Architecture® offers options that can redirect the focus from sexual pleasure if you need. In the following chapters, in addition to suggestions for improving sexual arousal, you'll also receive guidance on distinctive nervous system regulators for finding resiliency or joy related to each dimension.

While sexual pleasure might be a large part of some people's arousal system, it's not the whole picture. The Arousal Architecture® is based on more than just sexual context, and these resiliency tools or aspects of yourself can lead to sexual arousal and pleasure.

For example, your core values or values you desire in another partner can be a part of your Arousal Architecture® design. On dating site profiles, I've seen religious preferences or phrases that explain someone's political leanings, which might indicate a desire for a potential partner to align with them on topics like raising kids, social justice, or war. These values might fit into the

Embodied Experience and Energetic Connection dimensions. Folks find "non-sexual" stimulation (like values or political beliefs) just as relevant as if they're physically attracted to a partner.

These concepts are crucial to understand because they reveal there are so many more contributors to sexual arousal and pleasurable sex than we have been told to believe. Folks have thought that just because they're not turned on in "typical ways," something's wrong with them. Nothing could be further from the truth. We need to disrupt this belief system. Sexual pleasure and sexual arousal look different for everyone. So, we need to give ourselves compassion and grace when it doesn't look like the "standard" sexual response. It's time to find liberation by embracing what works for you!

#5 Arousal Architecture® Creates Opportunities for "Small Wins" to Rewire for Pleasure

You've been learning and applying the compound effect. Hopefully, you'll soon feel the benefits of implementing small, consistent changes in nervous system regulation and pleasure-building. Regularly practicing these "low-pressure" interventions creates a template (or collection of brain pathways), increasing familiarity with those skills and confidence in "high-pressure" situations (like sexual experiences). If you haven't already practiced them with sexual play, the Arousal Architecture® will provide you with opportunities to apply your newfound skills. Additionally, the Arousal Architecture® model might uncover options for more "small wins" with new thoughts or behaviors to enhance sexual resiliency.

Plus, when you use small-scale and easily attainable tools to experience success, you obtain immediate feedback that you know how to take control back over your body and influence it in a more regulated and resilient way. These increased abilities paired with nervous system awareness and regulation quickly lead to sexual arousal and confidence.

Remember, the aim is to rewrite your sexual narrative. The intentional structure of the Arousal Architecture® and the lessons within it are vital ways to continue creating new pathways for expanding your sexual satisfaction.

The Arousal Architecture® Assessment

Below are fifty questions asking about various situations mostly related to arousal and sexual situations. Although the Arousal Architecture® design can be used to reveal pleasure that isn't explicitly sexual, this is the starting point we're using for now.

Respond to the questions below to the best of your ability, answering "Mostly True" or "Mostly False." There's no right or wrong answer—only data!

Even if a question doesn't seem to fit you, trust that it's intentionally designed to provide you with the most sophisticated and personalized results. If you lean slightly toward one response, even if that's one degree, choose the option you're leaning toward. You'll be able to explore deeper into why you chose it later and in what situations it might be the other option.

Then, count the number of "Mostly True" responses for each dimension. This is your value for that dimension. Keep your final numbers and responses handy since you'll use them in the following chapters, as we discussed.

Sexual Stimulation

1. When I see my partner's (or someone's) naked body or parts of their body, I usually have pleasant sexual thoughts, feelings, or responses.
2. Watching porn or looking at explicit or pornographic images typically can stir something pleasant in me.
3. I like (or think I might like) to read or listen to erotica or stories about sexual situations.

4. Typically, when I watch a movie that has a sex scene in it, I find it pleasurable.

5. When my partner stimulates my genitals, it can turn me on "relatively" quickly.

6. When a sexual or romantic partner suggests that we should have sex, it is generally easy for me to get in the mood, too.

7. When my partner and I make out, it is usually easy enough for me to transition into other sexual play.

8. Experiencing orgasm is not usually a challenge for me.

9. I enjoy that sex often provides me an opportunity for pleasure or orgasm.

10. Most of the time, my body responds pleasantly to sexual situations, feelings, thoughts, or behaviors.

Total of "Mostly True" responses for Sexual Stimulation: _____

Embodied Experience

1. Before I can get in the mood, I need to feel physically safe and protected.

2. When my body feels uncomfortable or in pain, I cannot (or don't want to) engage in sexual play.

3. I really like to feel my lover stroke my hair and "traditionally" non-sexual parts of my body or hold me before I can even begin to feel a desire for sex.

4. If I don't exercise or meditate regularly, it's hard for me to relax enough to be sexual.

5. Dancing or other movements with my body help me feel sexy.

6. The smell of my partner's skin (or their other scents) makes me feel good and can even turn me on.

7. Skin-on-skin contact (either my partner's or my own) really helps me relax and can even turn me on.

8. To let go and be sexual, it often feels necessary to be in a room that is set up in a certain way for sexual play (e.g., it's tidy, the temperature is comfortable, or it has pleasant lighting).

9. The taste of my partner's skin or kiss is very pleasurable to me, and I can focus on pleasure when I think about how they taste.

10. Often, when I feel the pressure of my partner's body against or on me, I feel present and might have pleasurable sexual thoughts or feelings.

Total of "Mostly True" responses for Embodied Experience: _____

Mental Headspace

1. I find intellectually stimulating conversations enjoyable and they might even arouse me.

2. I need to know I am in a situation where I can express myself accurately and ask for what I need to feel at ease, especially to become aroused.

3. Sexy music helps me stay present, and if good jams are on, I can consider getting in the mood.

4. When my partner and I fight, I need things to feel resolved before I can engage in sexual play with them.

5. More times than not, if I'm too stressed, I can't even begin to think about sexual pleasure, let alone getting turned on.

6. I usually can't get in the mood if I know I must have a difficult conversation with my partner or someone else.

7. Typically, I have to know if my sexual partner has been tested for sexually transmitted infections (STDs/STIs) before I engage in "risky" sexual activity with them.

8. If I don't feel heard or respected by my partner, it's hard for me to desire to be close or sexual with them.

9. When I accomplish something important or my partner acknowledges my intellectual side, I feel excited or even turned on.

10. When I feel focused or organized in my life, it's easier for me to access sexual thoughts, desires, or feelings.

Total of "Mostly True" responses for Mental Headspace: _____

Energetic Connection

1. Typically, I have to know my partner well to engage in sexual activity with them.

2. When I feel like my partner "gets me," I might have a desire for sexual intimacy.

3. When I feel connected to spirituality (however I define that), I feel energized or might even be able to feel turned on.

4. Romantic experiences or gestures (e.g., date nights, gifts, or love letters) turn me on or help me feel closer to my partner.

5. When my values align with my partner, this makes me happy or even turned on.

6. When my partner demonstrates a commitment to me (and our family, if we have one), I feel more sexually or intimately available.

7. When I can express vulnerabilities (or my partner expresses theirs), I can feel a pull toward them or even be turned on by this.

8. When I feel connected to my sense of purpose, I can more easily access sexual thoughts, feelings, or desires.

9. It usually turns me on when my partner touches me in a way that seems to express their love or care for me.

10. I enjoy casual sex if I believe we have a good connection or we are aligned in our relational desires.

Total of "Mostly True" responses for Energetic Connection: _____

Erotic Exploration

1. I like the idea of a partner acting in a dominating (or submissive) way, sexually or otherwise.

2. I have had sexual fantasies that I would like to try out one day.

3. I feel ashamed of, embarrassed by, or guilty about something that turns me on.

4. I enjoy engaging in activities where I can get into a flow state or invest in exciting passion projects.

5. It turns me on when I think about using restraints (either giving or receiving) for sexual pleasure.

6. I have had sexual thoughts or desires about situations that might not be considered society's version of "normal."

7. I have had something unpleasant or significant happen to me in the past that is likely getting in the way of me being sexual or becoming turned on.

8. I like the idea of sexual role-play with my partner or in my fantasies.

9. When my partner and I are creative or playful together, I'm much more willing to be sexually engaged and explorative.

10. I enjoy trying new things sexually, even if that means I might be a little uncomfortable or awkward doing it—the payoff likely means that I find something new to turn me on.

Total of "Mostly True" responses for Erotic Exploration: _____

9

The Sexual Stimulation Dimension

In case it's not apparent, the Sexual Stimulation dimension includes the importance of explicitly sexual stimuli or contexts in your Arousal Architecture®. These stimuli are expressive sexual actions, thoughts, feelings, and desires. Most people would objectively agree that these experiences are typically considered sexually arousing or "turn-ons." This dimension tells us how influential straightforward sexual acts are in helping you become aroused.

Folks who find this dimension resonant enjoy thinking about sexual contexts and engaging in sexual play (depending on how someone defines "sex"). Further, people who connect with the Sexual Stimulation dimension often have a version of their sex life that they feel relatively good about or feel sexually satisfied. Being sexual might be a part of their usual routine, whether that's with masturbation, thoughts, or sex with others. Their sexuality is a part of who they are, even if they want to improve their sex life.

On-ramps for the Sexual Stimulation dimension are attraction and sexual openness. Off-ramps are pretty much everything you've read in the book, such as stress, discomfort, unpleasant experiences, or emotions. Your on- and off-ramps might differ from someone else's and fluctuate depending on mood, partners, or stressors.

Sexual Stimulation Dimension Examples

- The physical appearance of a partner.
- Genital stimulation.
- Porn, erotica, or romance novels that focus on frequent and steamy sex scenes.
- Intense kissing.
- Wearing lingerie or seeing a partner wear lingerie.
- Knowing you'll meet with a partner later and that you'll engage in sexual play.
- Fantasizing about someone or a sexual situation you would like to happen.

What Your Dimension Total Reveals About Your Arousal Language

Total = 6+

If your level of Sexual Stimulation dimension is 6 or higher, then you probably respond pleasantly to straightforward sexual stimulation and find sexual energy, interactions, or contexts enjoyable and accessible. You likely have a "spontaneous desire" and can easily anticipate pleasure, which leads to quicker sexual arousal. Also, you can likely reach orgasm without much effort.

Suppose your total is high (8–10), and most other dimensions are not. In that case, you can optimize your pleasure and arousal potentials in more areas of your life than explicitly sexual contexts by enhancing the other dimensions.

Total = 3–5

A number lower than 5 doesn't mean your sexual arousal is lacking; it simply suggests there are plenty of options to explore other dimensions. Lucky you! Let's hop on an adventure to find out how to discover them using the exercises that follow.

If your number is 3–5 and your other dimensions are much higher, you likely enjoy explicitly sexual stimulation when you've had time to "warm up," or you've been able to spend a solid amount of time getting your other needs met. This total reveals that you have a long on-ramp and responsive desire. There's absolutely nothing wrong with this. In fact, most of my clients find this assessment resonant and feel relieved knowing others do, too. The supplemental exercises and suggestions for the other dimensions of the Arousal Architecture® help them integrate their on-ramps more seamlessly into their lives. I hope you'll find empowerment knowing it is typical and perfectly sexy to need something different than what someone with spontaneous desire needs.

Total = 0–2

Explicit sexual acts might not be fundamental to arouse you, which implies different needs or approaches to access arousal before you can get in the mood (if that's what you even want). You're not alone in having a total of 0–2. Some people (for instance, asexual folks) find that explicitly sexual acts are not inviting and do not prefer to engage in them for their own arousal. And that's 1,000 percent okay!

This total implies that you would prefer a minimal focus on explicitly sexual acts and that your pleasure potential comes from one of the other dimensions. That's why Arousal Architecture® is so incredible! Many folks love learning how to prioritize those needs just as much as someone who has an arousal system with a higher desire for explicitly sexual acts in their lives.

If you have a total of 0 and are satisfied with it, that's amazing! Then, you may not want to explore this chapter further. However, it could be beneficial to learn about this dimension if it's essential to a partner.

Remember, we've been taught incorrectly about what pleasure and sexual arousal are and what is considered "normal." This misconception has caused many of us to feel terrible about something quite common and healthy.

Suggestions and Interventions for Sexual Stimulation Dimension

The following are tips and exercises to help you become more familiar with this aspect of your sexual self. Some can help you adjust your total if that's what you desire. Others will help you identify what you like to gain awareness of your arousal language and make it easier to share with others. You'll find the same structure in the following four chapters, so I won't repeat these instructions again to avoid redundancy.

Exercises for Optimizing Your Sexual Stimulation Dimension

- Create a "Sexual Menu."
    - You can do this by listing thoughts, behaviors, or contexts you know you find sexually pleasing. We started this process when you listed on-ramps in Chapter 7.
    - If you're having trouble thinking of possibilities or need more inspiration, you can respond to a "Yes, No, Maybe" List, which we'll discuss in Part 4.
    - Also, your Arousal Architecture® results will help you add to your Sexual Menu. As you work through each dimension, you'll find

more items to include that you wouldn't have previously thought were "sexual."

- Something in your Arousal Architecture® might start as a "non-sexual" behavior or thought (such as long, slow strokes on your back). Then, by using some of the exercises in this book, you create a brain pathway connecting sexually arousing sensations and associations to it. You could then update your Sexual Menu to incorporate those experiences.

- Use the Mirror Exercise from Chapter 6 to become more familiar with your genitals and parts for Pleasure Potential. Identify the places and kinds of touch you enjoy by exploring yourself. Add lube to the mix for better sensations and sexual health!

Want to Increase or Reduce Your Dimension Total?

The first part of this section provides considerations and interventions if your total is notably higher relative to the Embodied Experience, Mental Headspace, or Energetic Connection dimensions. This combination of totals implies you have many more possibilities to optimize your arousal and pleasure potential by tapping into the resources of the other dimensions.

Some situations might inspire you to reduce your number in this dimension if you feel concerned about how much you focus on explicitly sexual stimuli. For instance, if you're worried about your sexually compulsive tendencies or a partner mentions they need more time with their on-ramp, but you continue to engage in explicitly sexual stimuli. Further, it could be beneficial if you want to reduce your focus on orgasm and enjoy the journey more.

I want to clarify that I'm not suggesting that having a high total in this dimension is problematic. As with any of the dimensions, all that matters is the meaning you determine of your Arousal Architecture® results and what you decide aligns with your values and goals.

These interventions can help address a high total in this dimension, if you want to create more balance in your Arousal Architecture®. Many of these strategies are ones you've encountered before, which can provide a sense of familiarity and reassurance in your journey.

- Engage or review the Sexual Pleasure Paradigm Shift from Chapter 6.
- Explore your purpose for engaging in sex, as explained in Chapter 7.
- Build a Pleasurable Connection Beyond Your Genitals, as we explored in Chapter 6.
- Consider that a high focus on orgasm instead of also pleasure or connection is limiting your sexual satisfaction. Or that you define successful sexual outcomes based on how well your genitals "perform" (erection or lubrication) or if you or others have an orgasm.

The following are suggestions for folks who wish to build more access to the influence of the Sexual Stimulation dimension. Most of the book is about improving your sexual arousal system and sexual satisfaction (based on how you define "satisfying"). So, you can't go wrong with using any of the exercises we've explored already. Usually, the following are my starting points after creating a solid foundation (which is what you've been doing throughout this book).

- Notice the sensations in your body when you experience "non-sexual" pleasures and spend time savoring them. This will build more possibilities for pleasure pathways.
- Build Sexual Resiliency as discussed in Chapter 5 along with the effective communication tools in Part 4.
- Try the Breathe Out Anxiety, Breathe In Arousal exercise from Chapter 6.
  - This exercise will help you reduce distractions, anxiety, or thought spirals getting in your way of being present around sexual experiences.

- Engage in the exercise from Chapter 7: Connect Passionate Energy to Your Genitals.
  - This exercise can awaken sexual energy by using the template of noticing exciting energy from other aspects of your life to your sexual energy.
- Build confidence in skills or techniques for explicitly sexual experiences, such as taking local sex-positive adult education classes or online courses—you can find my favorites in the back of the book.
- Pelvic Pain Patients or Sexually Anxious Folks: Take the Arousal Architecture®; then, after working with a therapist or coach or engaging in your treatment recommendations (applying your prescribed creams, using your dilators, attending physical therapy, etc.), retake the Arousal Architecture® assessment and compare your results.

Exercises

Quick Win!

Identify your top three to five items in the Sexual Stimulation dimension. With these, you're starting your "Sexual Menu." Add any detail that feels relevant to your items.

Going Deeper

For a refresher on the detailed instructions, refer to the end of Chapter 8.

Reflect on your responses to the questions you had the strongest responses to when you answered. It doesn't matter if you responded, "Mostly True" or "Mostly False." Identify the details of your responses. Then, examine *why* you answered the way you did or interview yourself with the relevant questions from the "5W and H" journalism technique ("Who?" "What?" "Why?" etc.).

Below are some prompts to show you how to examine the responses in this dimension further. Use this as a guide for the other dimensions, too.

- What is it about sexually explicit stimuli (e.g., touch, context, thoughts, or behaviors) that you enjoy compared to what you do not find pleasurable?

- Do you enjoy porn or erotica because of who's involved or because of the context of the situation? *Interesting note*: Research shows that cis men or folks assigned male at birth tend to prefer the former, whereas cis women or folks assigned female at birth respond to the latter.[1]

- Are there certain parts of your body that you enjoy being touched or stimulated regardless of your level of perceived sexual arousal? What about when you psychologically desire sexual interaction even if your body hasn't shown signs of obvious sexual arousal? We're talking about arousal non-concordance, as we talked about in Chapter 6. You can watch a fantastic TED talk by Emily Nagoski about this, too.[2]

- Are there certain parts of your body you do not want to be touched until you feel sufficiently aroused or when you tell your partner(s) it's okay to touch them?

- Do you know a timeframe that you typically need or desire for sensual touching, kissing, or other similar activities before you are ready to engage in something more explicit? Remember, it could be a minute or forty minutes—there's no right or wrong, only preferences!

10

The Embodied Experience Dimension

I know, I know. Being "embodied" is a buzzword right now and can even sound a little "woo." You might imagine some light-energized yoga instructor discussing getting "in your body." To be totally honest, that's how I was initially introduced to the concept. As a perfectionist living primarily "in my head" and not knowing what it meant to be embodied, I thought achieving it was impossible. Then, I dove into the science of it all and became certified in somatic trauma treatment. I learned it was not only a powerful healing modality but also essential for sexual and overall wellness.

As a reminder, being embodied means bringing awareness to the present moment and being aware of your body, needs, energy levels, and moods. Mindfulness is an aspect of being embodied. Living as an embodied person can be difficult, particularly if you've had sexual challenges, need to manage pain, or deal with overwhelming stressors of life.

It's a simple enough concept to understand that an embodied life is vital to wellness, but applying it to your life can feel complicated. That's why Embodied Experience gets its own dimension in the Arousal Architecture®. This dimension can be crucial to unlocking arousal and pleasure potential if you struggle with anxious or painful sex. It's also potent for optimizing sexual experiences and quality of life.

The Embodied Experience dimension aims to create awareness around your sexual, psychological, and energetic needs through the mind-body connection. It further aims to identify the contexts, thoughts, and behaviors that help you feel more regulated and "in your body" in sexual situations as well as life experiences.

Our bodies are intricate and complex machines. However, this is wildly simple: if the body is not taken care of, the other systems, like the sexual arousal system, will not operate well either. On-ramps for the Embodied Experience dimension are body-centered and grounded experiences, while the off-ramps are usually situations that create a state of disconnection from your body.

Embodied Experience Dimension Examples

Remember, the total number is how influential this dimension is to create arousal. You might see some examples below and know they would likely apply to everyone (like "physical safety" for instance). However, it's not that you do or don't want Embodied Experiences in your life. Instead, it's about how *crucial* these contexts are for you to access joy, sexual arousal, and pleasure.

- Physical safety (or at least risk-aware and consensual agreements of potential physical danger, such as in BDSM [bondage and discipline, dominance and submission, sadism and masochism] activities).
- Not experiencing sexual pain or discomfort.
- A beautiful space or ambiance.
- Pleasant scents or how a partner smells.
- Engaging in an activity that feels energizing instead of depleting.
- Engaging in mindfulness, meditation, or regular exercise that helps you feel grounded or energized.

- Non-genital touch that feels soothing, comforting, or enjoyable.
- Porn, erotica, or romance novels that include humor, lightness, and body positivity.

What Your Dimension Total Reveals About Your Arousal Language

Total = 6+

Let's say you have a high number in the Embodied Experience dimension. In that case, when your body feels comfortable, at peace, relaxed, safe, and pain-free (or reduced pain), it has a significant impact on your sexual arousal system. Alternatively, if you don't feel good in or connected to your body, it can be difficult to enjoy an experience and even more challenging to become aroused. Prioritizing your self-care needs outside of the metaphorical bedroom can help you enjoy what goes on *in* the bedroom.

The Mindfulness, Somatics, and Your Brain chapters might resonate with you, so revisiting those concepts can help you create a better connection to your body in neutral or pleasant ways. Setting the mood could also be essential for you—the proper lighting, room temperature, or pleasant smells can set the stage for your nervous system to settle and access arousal. You're not alone in this—a research study found that "mood setting" was a crucial factor in keeping passion alive![1]

A high number in this dimension with low numbers in Sexual Stimulation or Erotic Exploration could reveal that you have responsive desire. A high total while experiencing sexual challenges could also indicate that your needs for arousal are not prioritized as much as you need or as your partner's. You might also not even know what you want or need to access your arousal yet. Allow yourself to embrace a longer on-ramp and celebrate that "warming up" is paramount to your sexual arousal system and pleasure.

Total = 0–5

A lower total in the Embodied Experience dimension implies that it's not as necessary to focus on embodiment to easily access arousal. It doesn't mean that you are "disembodied" (or detached from your body) sexually. Instead, it suggests it's not an essential aspect to reach sexual arousal.

However, if you have difficulties with sex, arousal, and pleasure, it implies you don't connect with your body enough to achieve the levels of sexual wellness or satisfaction you desire. The interventions below can increase body awareness and mindfulness, leading to a more satisfying (sex) life.

Generally, the idea is to create "body safety." You can do this in various ways, some overlapping significantly with the other dimensions. Being embodied is a core need for healthy sexuality. I always encourage embodiment as a wellness skill for overall life satisfaction, so this dimension can be an area to expand upon constantly. Doing so can lead to a happier life and deeper, more powerful pleasure and orgasms!

Suggestions and Interventions for Embodied Experience Dimension

The overall goal of the Embodied Experience dimension is to expand resiliency. Almost anything discussed in this book can facilitate being more embodied. Below, you'll find my favorite recommendations to cultivate more embodied experiences and optimize your sex life and beyond.

Exercises for Optimizing Your Embodied Experience Dimension

- Intentionally practice self-care in ways that make sense for you, whether with a massage, setting boundaries, or something else entirely.

- Regularly use somatic exercises as discussed in Chapter 3. Remember to use them in sexual situations as well.

- Notice pleasant sensations, as we explored in Chapter 3. Spend the day noticing them. Focus on pleasant sensations when engaging in sex.

- Identify sexual thoughts, scenarios, or contexts that help you feel good in your body, then do more of them. Identify the ones that do not and limit those.

Want to Increase or Reduce Your Dimension Total?

It feels counterintuitive to suggest options to reduce the influence of the Embodied Experience dimension. It might only be an issue if you're unsatisfied with your Arousal Architecture® results and find that this is the highest or one of your only high totals. Still, I recommend increasing the other dimensions before decreasing this one.

Similar issues can cause your total to be high or low. So, I will combine the interventions for this dimension because they apply to any total amount.

The first circumstance I'll point out is for high-achievers, perfectionists, or people-pleasers who overwork or focus more on others' needs while typically neglecting their own. Let's say this resonates with you. Since you can't pour from an empty cup, you will ultimately feel depleted or burnt out if you don't prioritize your needs. You've likely heard to "do more self-care" from doctors, social media, partners, or friends, and we often think it refers to more bubble baths, massages, or vacations. While those can be helpful, it's essential to consider self-care in the form of setting boundaries or asking for what you want or need. A low mind-body connection can make it difficult even to be aware that you're burning out. You also may not know what you need or when you need it. In that case, the Arousal Architecture® is valuable because it helps you identify action items to learn what you enjoy.

Those situations can relate to sexual contexts as well. The pressure of sexual performance (such as engaging in sexual activities for your partner's benefit and not prioritizing your own) is a quick path to disembodiment.

Remember that you don't need an elaborate self-care routine. I don't know about you, but my clients and I are busy and sometimes can't even squeeze in ten minutes for self-care practices or meditation. I've developed a unique ability to help active folks like executives, parents, teachers, lawyers, students, and healthcare providers find interventions that fit even the busiest schedules. Finding practical exercises that are easy to remember and slip into your daily routine without added burden is crucial. Hopefully, some of what you've read in this book can help you identify the interventions that work well for you.

Another situation where the Embodied Experience interventions can be helpful is if you experience a lot of physical pain (like fibromyalgia, vaginismus, or endometriosis) or emotional pain (such as trauma, sexual challenges, or body image concerns). Being embodied can feel incredibly threatening because it can exacerbate your experience of pain. However, the goal of the interventions here is to be aware and mindful in ways that interrupt the threat response, help you feel empowered, and effectively down-regulate your nervous system more effectively. Focus on using tools that gradually help you feel more in control of your body and emotions such as mindfulness, somatic interventions, or those explained in the rest of the book. While nervous system regulation is useful for all dimensions, it's imperative in the Embodied Experience.

The following are my favorite recommendations if you are not satisfied with your sex life or want to improve it using Embodied Experience exercises. While I can't say that the exercises that follow will fit perfectly for you, they can be a starting point. Get creative about how to incorporate them into your life!

- Regularly engage in mindfulness or somatic practices to regulate your nervous system, such as the practices you resonated with in Chapters 2 or 3.

- Use the exercise Breathe Out Anxiety, Breathe In Arousal as described in Chapter 6.
- Set healthy boundaries and be compassionate with yourself about doing so.
- Identify off-ramps and on-ramps related to your physical comfort.

Exercises

Quick Win!

List three to five conditions or situations that make being intimate or sexual feel good for your body. Describe the scenarios in detail, if you wish.

Going Deeper

For a refresher on the detailed instructions, refer to the end of Chapter 8.
Reflect on your responses to the Arousal Architecture® questions you most reacted to when you answered. Expand your understanding of the details of your responses by examining *why* you answered the way you did. Dive into the meanings or significance of the questions and your responses by using the "5W and H" journalism technique.

11

The Mental Headspace Dimension

The Mental Headspace dimension relates to how influential your state of mind is in achieving arousal and pleasure. It can also reflect the need to regulate your mind and mental wellness, especially in sexual or romantic situations. Someone who resonates with this dimension might describe themselves as being "in their head" often or having a lot of stress. This dimension can assist you in finding ways to engage or utilize your mind for mental health, attraction, or sexual arousal.

Folks relying on cognitive processes and logical problem-solving over feelings and emotions enjoy using the Mental Headspace dimension's exercises and interventions. Structure and organization can almost be a turn-on, and even if not, those qualities can at least provide a container that makes it easier to access arousal and pleasure. Using their mind's abilities helps them feel grounded and safe. While the Embodied Experience dimension focuses on creating safety in the body, the Mental Headspace dimension concentrates on building a psychological or cognitive sense of safety and resiliency.

If you resonate with this dimension, you probably enjoyed learning about the ideas in the Mindset, Your Brain, and Your Energy chapters. You might have a job or hobby that relies heavily on your cognitive capabilities. Your friendships and other relationships presumably focus on sharing ideas, analyzing concepts, or planning.

Connecting with a partner on a cognitive level or engaging in activities facilitating captivating conversations could be critical contributors to your Mental Headspace. Addressing concerns or conversations about where the relationship stands, sexually transmitted infection testing or status, or future relationship preferences or plans utilizes the power of this dimension.

As an example, folks in the LGBTQ+, poly, or kink communities might be at a different stage than their partner(s) regarding coming out to their straight, monogamous, or vanilla friends and family. Discussing the differences among partners and determining how to navigate them are necessary for all parties to feel heard, respected, and cared for. This commitment reflects respect for their mental or intellectual safety of the Mental Headspace dimension, which optimizes intimacy, sexual arousal, pleasure, and satisfaction.

Even folks not in those communities benefit from effective communication about relationship expectations. In a study of over 38,000 people, participants in long-term monogamous committed relationships reported that communication about sex and the relationship was associated with higher levels of relationship and sexual satisfaction.[1] As such, it makes sense that knowing and expressing needs regarding the relationship or sex can relieve tension in the nervous system.

Mental stress or lack of clarity can create off-ramps for sexual experiences. On the other hand, talking about sex, managing stress, and stimulating the mind are all powerful tenets of the Mental Headspace dimension. These tenets create potent on-ramps for folks who resonate with this dimension.

Remember that your total does not mean your results indicate anything positive or negative about this dimension. Instead, focus on which aspects of your Mental Headspace are influential and why. Also, remember that contributors to this dimension aren't limited to sexual or relationship needs; they can also relate to your overall mental well-being.

Mental Headspace Dimension Examples

- Playing cards or strategy board games.
- The ability to have healthy communication and understanding with others.
- Having a calm or quiet mind or using stress-management techniques.
- Determining and asserting boundaries (notice this can be in multiple dimensions).
- Knowing and communicating about your hard limits, soft limits, and negotiables for sexual play.
- Porn, erotica, or romance novels that pair sexual energy with witty dialogue (the Netflix series, *Bridgerton*, anyone?).
- Identifying and committing to an aftercare plan for BDSM (bondage and discipline, dominance and submission, sadism and masochism) or sexual play activities.

What Your Dimension Total Reveals About Your Arousal Language

Total = 6+

Typically, people who identify as sapiosexuals, academics, business owners, executives, and neurodivergent folks have high levels in the Mental Dimension. It also relates well to those often "in their heads" and who need distractions from worries to access arousal.

If you have a high total, you might feel overstimulated with many choices or "noise" in your mind, such as anxiety, stressors, performance concerns, or fears. Doing what you can to quiet them down is crucial for your arousal needs.

A high number in the Mental Headspace dimension might mean you enjoy or have an exceptional "mental game" when it comes to sexual arousal, such as erotic stories or dirty talk. Being a heady person, you enjoy stimulating your brain as much as your body. Enjoyable conversations contribute to your on-ramp toward sexual arousal or play. Prioritizing core values, aligning with belief systems, or having similar perspectives on life or sex will likely be turn-ons.

Dealing with sexual challenges and having a high total in the Mental Headspace dimension could signify a struggle to turn your brain off or focus on your present experience. Sexual performance issues, life or relationship uncertainties, and expectations are common complaints for folks who lean toward this dimension.

Total = 0–5

Having a lower total here can reveal that your mind is not necessarily a key to turning you on. You might be a person who can quickly turn off "internal chatter" in sexual situations. This skill can be a very effective way to manage stress and have satisfying sexual experiences. Also, you might not need to know the meaning or timeline of the relationship. You can be content with experiencing it as it is without it bothering you.

A low total in the Mental Headspace could be problematic if you find that you're not intentional enough in the conversations you have around sex or relationships. You might find that you deal with situations as they arise instead of being communicative in advance or expressing what you genuinely want. Suppose you have sexual challenges and a low number in this dimension. In that case, you might feel unsure or apathetic about your arousal or relationships, deferring to others' preferences. It could indicate a low mood, depression, or feeling stuck in life. Lacking a sense of purpose or meaning can also contribute to sexual challenges, as we explored in Chapter 7.

Suggestions and Interventions for Mental Headspace Dimension

Exercises for Optimizing Your Mental Headspace Dimension

- Use practical communication tools to express what you want and need such as with those found in Part 4.
- Listen to audio erotica or read romance novels with strong, determined characters you can identify with. It's also helpful if the stories are written well or have engaging or complex scenarios.
- Engage in dirty talk or ask a partner to. There's a guide on How to Talk Dirty in Part 4!
- Use mindfulness strategies before, during, and after sexual play.
- Commit to living by your core values.
- Identify thought processes that help you stay present and focused.

Want to Increase or Reduce Your Dimension Total?

Similar to the Embodied Experience dimension, the interventions can overlap. You might not want to reduce your total and instead prefer to manage it with the interventions. The aim is to create resources for a mental landscape stimulated by titillating mental experiences while remaining relaxed and resilient.

- Identify any Limiting Beliefs you still might have. Then, rewrite them as you did in Chapter 4.
- Engage in the Cognitive and Somatic Reframe for limiting thoughts or beliefs, as explained in Chapter 6.
- Use the Compassionate Script from Chapter 4 when you notice critical self-talk arising.

- Engage in effective communication strategies (such as the interventions you'll find in Part 4).
- Seek a sex-positive therapist to explore the cognitive processes that seem to get in your way of a more fulfilled life and satisfying sex life.

Exercises

Quick Win!

Identify your top three to five ideal Mental Headspace experiences with as much detail as you can or desire.

Going Deeper

For a refresher on the detailed instructions, refer to the end of Chapter 8.
Reflect on your responses to the Arousal Architecture® questions you most reacted to, then examine *why* you answered the way you did.

12

The Energetic Connection Dimension

The Energetic Connection dimension relates to the emotional, energetic, or intimate connection someone needs for arousal. This dimension can be about an energetic or intimate connection with oneself or another person.

Within a partnership, the Energetic Connection dimension focuses on emotional investment and intentional attachment to each other. Typically, romance, sensuality, or respect govern these kinds of interactions. Also, people who find this dimension resonant prefer some level of closeness before they can access arousal or engage in sex. Being told how much they are wanted, loved, or cared for matters significantly to them. Sensual kissing, touching, or embracing often enough lights a sexual spark for someone who finds the Energetic Connection dimension influential. These folks are initially more interested in and aroused by the dynamic of the characters in porn, erotica, or romance stories than the sex acts or characters themselves. However, once they have the juicy context of the characters and the relationship between them, watch out—things will get steamy rapidly!

This dimension is not limited to partnerships. Folks can fill their energetic cup through their internal connection to themselves, their experience of accomplishment (however that looks), or a sense of self-worth.

Some people feel inspired or regulated by their spiritual or religious connections, which can facilitate a portion of their Energetic Connection. If that's the case for you, it can support a resilient mind and body, opening more possibilities for arousal. Even if you're not spiritual, this dimension still relates to how you feel about yourself and your commitment to your needs, interests, and life overall.

This dimension focuses on creating energetic safety through connection and compassion. It's the epitome of intimacy. Most people use the term "intimacy" as a euphemism for sexual activities. Instead, intimacy (particularly in this context) refers to a deep closeness, especially in vulnerable ways.

Although most people understand intimacy in the context of certain types of committed and monogamous relationships, intimacy can also be a part of casual sexual relationships, BDSM (bondage and discipline, dominance and submission, sadism and masochism) play partners, and consensually non-monogamous dynamics. These styles of relationships might not expect emotional dependence beyond the boundaries of the relationship. Yet, they can still feel intimately satisfied with them, utilizing the power of the Energetic Connection dimension.

For instance, think about someone so focused on their career that they do not want to prioritize seriously committed relationships and the required time or energy. Still, they enjoy having meaningful sex, flirty involvements, or friends with benefits. They are not flippant about the other person's emotions or needs. As long as all parties agree on the expectations for the relationship, it can remain non-committal while still intimate or energetically connected.

Another example is a "unicorn" (a person who joins a couple, either sexually or romantically). All three people can engage in intimate or deep connections. However, the unicorn might not have the same level of emotional interdependence as the couple does to each other by design.

Intimacy doesn't have to relate to committed relationships or even romance. You can find it in friendships, role models, therapists, and even simply knowing yourself.

If the Energetic Connection dimension resonates with you, you probably enjoyed the content in Chapter 7. Closeness, sensuality, romance, or personal power are the usual on-ramps for energetic connection. Off-ramps could include carelessness in relationships, distance, or resentment.

Remember, although the Arousal Architecture® is to help you engage your sexual arousal system, it doesn't mean that the path to arousal starts with sexual topics or content. It begins with a regulated nervous system along with your unique arousal language. Intentional energetic connections can increase resilience and authentic arousal significantly.

Energetic Connection Dimension Examples

- Emotional availability and intelligence.
- Tender sensuality, such as soft touch, strokes, embracing each other, and giving or receiving massages.
- Having a special spiritual connection within yourself or to something else energetically larger than you.
- Individual autonomy while remaining connected.
- Erotica, porn, or romance novels focusing on forbidden love, romantic suspense, or intimate relationships (*Bridgerton* for the win, again).
- Strong sense of self-worth.

What Your Dimension Total Reveals About Your Arousal Language

Total = 6+

A high number in the Energetic Connection dimension reveals that your arousal potential significantly depends on connected and invested experiences with others or a sense of connection to yourself. High totals could also emphasize the importance of deeper intimacy needs, which is a beautiful way to experience closeness and sexual interactions with your partner or yourself. Vulnerability and closeness are something you value and can be vital in turning you on.

You would benefit from longer on-ramps or more time to warm up. Often, your primary motivation for engaging in sexual play is intimacy with your partner. To feel sufficiently aroused or sexually satisfied, an emotionally available partner who's willing to commit to similar levels can be crucial for you.

Additionally, you likely relish deep connections with others in platonic ways, such as in friendships or with your family. Further, investing in self-love, valuing commitments you make to yourself, and finding pride in what you do fuel the Energetic Connection dimension. These situations can help facilitate life satisfaction and possibly inspire sexual satisfaction.

Some folks only desire intimate or emotional connection within a relationship without sex or with limited amounts of it, which is perfectly acceptable!

Now, let's say you're not interested in committed monogamous partnerships. In that case, consensually non-monogamous dynamics might only suit you if they feel meaningful and emotionally available, even in a limited dynamic.

Sexual challenges that coincide with high Energetic Connection dimension totals could signify dissatisfaction in the relationship, over-dependency on others (some call it co-dependence, but I'm not a fan of the stigma associated with that term), or low self-esteem. It might also indicate a heavier prioritization of your partner's pleasure. Additionally, imbalances in the relationship as it relates to taking care of the home, childcare, or emotional labor can create low arousal and reduced sexual satisfaction.

Total = 0–5

If you have a low number here, it doesn't mean you don't seek intimacy or connection with your partner. Instead, vulnerability or closeness is less critical to you than the stimulation from other dimensions for your arousal or pleasure potential. Also, a low number could reflect that an energetic connection with yourself or something spiritual is not necessarily part of your sexual self.

A low total in the Energetic Connection dimension could refer to a desire for casual relationships or sexual dynamics that don't depend on emotional availability or investment. This relationship preference doesn't imply a lack of care for partners as human beings. Instead, it suggests that committed or emotional investment is not a primary motivation for you to achieve arousal or sexual satisfaction.

However, if you have a low total in the Energetic Connection dimension and sexual challenges, it could indicate intimacy barriers, self-esteem challenges, or minimal spiritual connections (however you define them).

Suggestions and Interventions for Energetic Connection Dimension

Exercises for Optimizing Your Energetic Connection Dimension

Research shows that higher levels of emotional intimacy or intelligence create more opportunities for sexual satisfaction in most folks and relationship styles (monogamous compared to consensually non-monogamous), regardless of sexual orientation.[1] The following suggestions can help you access the power of the Energetic Connection dimension for yourself or within any relational dynamic.

- Schedule opportunities for intimacy. Really. Put time in the calendar to connect with yourself or your partner. Focus on emotional connection and joy while removing pressure on sex or orgasm, as discussed in Chapter 7.

- Embrace your off- and on-ramps!

- Engage in sensual play before other kinds of sex.

- Write a Love Letter to yourself or your partner, or ask your partner to write one for you (see Chapter 15).

- Engage in flirting or courting—refer to the How to Flirt guide in Chapter 15 for ideas!

Want to Increase or Reduce Your Dimension Total?

Like the Embodied Experience and Mental Headspace dimensions, I typically recommend helping folks embrace the influence of the Energetic Connection dimension if they have a high total.

In instances with low sexual arousal or satisfaction, it's necessary to understand why the levels are high and what's causing the sexual challenges. While we wouldn't likely concentrate on reducing the total in this dimension, you might consider how to meet your energetic, emotional, or intimate needs differently.

Regardless of your total in the Energetic Connection dimension, the following exercises can help you find greater satisfaction, arousal, and pleasure if you're struggling.

- Attend couples or sex therapy with a sex-positive somatic therapist.

- Explore intimacy barriers around giving or receiving vulnerable connection or love.

- Identify challenges with embracing self-love.

- Practice Sensate Focus.
  - While the traditional version of Sensate Focus may not be suitable for everyone, rest assured that alternative methods are available. I

teach an adapted version based on the NeuroSomaticSex Method™. If this is not accessible to you, there are sex therapists who can guide you through Sensate Focus effectively.

- Identify and discuss any imbalances in the relationship and your arousal needs with your partner.

Exercises

Quick Win!

Identify your top three to five Energetic Connection experiences and provide details to expand on their meaning and the conditions in which they would ideally happen.

Going Deeper

For a refresher on the detailed instructions, refer to the end of Chapter 8.
Reflect on your responses to the Arousal Architecture® questions you most reacted to when you answered. Dive into the meanings or significance of the questions and your responses by examining *why* you answered the way you did.

13

The Erotic Exploration Dimension

The Erotic Exploration dimension for sexual arousal encompasses aspects of arousal and sexual experiences that push up against the edge of expectation, excitement, or society's understanding of "typical." There can be a wide range of aspects to the Erotic Exploration dimension, from something as "mild" as trying new sexual positions to the "wild," such as engaging in sexual fetishes or BDSM (bondage and discipline, dominance and submission, sadism and masochism). Elements of this dimension might extend into or combine anything from intense eroticism to playful to "weird."

Don't get me wrong. I love weird and non-typical things. In fact, a component of my sexual healing and strength came from embracing what felt like "shameful secrets" that society deemed "not normal." On my healing journey, I accepted my authentic arousal and pleasure needs. By challenging societal expectations, I took control of my sexuality and liberated myself from those constraints. It was empowering and life-changing since it was essential in resolving sexual pain, too. My sexual narrative was my own, and I sought out people and partners who celebrated me for me.

Although I've embraced the word "weird," for some folks, it can still hold a stigma. So, instead, I'll use "edgy" as an umbrella term for everything within the Erotic Exploration dimension. One of the main goals of this book and the

Arousal Architecture® is to normalize all consensual sexual acts, desires, and relationship dynamics. I value breaking stigmas that are often associated with consensual and unconventional sexual desires or behaviors.

A significant part of my transformation wasn't just about embracing edgy sexual interests; it was also about everything discussed in this book—challenging expectations and belief systems around perfectionism, traditional gender roles, and productivity culture, for example. My point is that my "edgy" can be completely different from your "edgy," and it doesn't have to relate to sex at all.

I'm not suggesting that the Erotic Exploration dimension is about getting kinky. Instead, it's about celebrating the parts of you that you desire that have felt unjustly shameful or embarrassing. For example, it could be about having sex in the living room when the kids are at school or wearing more revealing clothing for date night than you typically would. One of my clients was thrilled to start buying clothes and painting her nails in ways that made her feel sexy and erotic instead of her usual "cute" or "pretty." She came from a family and community steeped in purity culture. After achieving pain-free sex and releasing sexual shame, she and her partner embraced fun and erotic explorations, optimizing their sex life in ways that worked for them and their belief systems.

Let's take a moment to understand what "erotic" means and how it's different from "sexual," at least regarding the Arousal Architecture®. The Oxford Language definition of erotic is "relating to or tending to arouse sexual desire or excitement," which doesn't quite capture it for me.

However, I'm obsessed with the marvelous Audre Lorde's conceptualization of eroticism. She coined the idea of "the erotic" in her essay, "Uses of the Erotic: The Erotic as Power."[1] Lorde explained that "the erotic offers a well of replenishing and provocative force to the woman who does not fear its revelation, nor succumb to the belief that sensation is enough." In the essay, Lorde continues to explore the concept that denying erotic power is the effort of an oppressive culture aiming to control sexuality and women (and, in my modern opinion, all genders striving to break free of conventional expectations of sexual behavior and wellness). Beyond sexual energy, Lorde also explores the potent force of erotic power to encourage seeking excellence in life without demanding the impossible. She claims we can transform our lives through intentional decisions that bring us closer to rejuvenating fullness.

As such, eroticism is about a vitality or an energy force for sexually enticing thoughts, contexts, or behaviors that can incorporate mental, embodied, and energetic experiences. Essentially, it can combine some or all of the Arousal Architecture® dimensions. This integration is why most items you discover about yourself in the other dimensions could overlap in the Erotic Exploration dimension with some creative plotting (which I love doing). Erotic Exploration goes beyond elemental sexual energy; it captures the internal passionate quality of what makes each of us light up with desire (sexually or otherwise).

The Erotic Exploration dimension is about adventure, connection, and a desire to push against the edge of comfort to optimize your pleasure (in all forms) and sex life. Kinky activities and BDSM are perfect examples of the Erotic Exploration dimension. As researchers so aptly put it, BDSM "can be understood as a process of increasing expansion, creation, and connection, in which desire is seen not as something we lack or need, but rather as a process of striving and self-enhancement."

You don't have to be kinky or into BDSM to unlock the power of exploring eroticism, as there are many more ways to tap into erotic energy beyond those. I reference BDSM because research is uncovering that "kink sexuality can be an opportunity for peoples' personal growth, self-actualization, healing, and transformation."[2] One study found that BDSM practitioners were less neurotic and rejection sensitive. They were also more extroverted, open to new experiences, conscientious, and had higher subjective well-being than the control groups.[3] Not everyone would identify themselves as kinky, but after twenty years of being in the field and asking people what kind of sexual play they like, a lot of folks end up describing something that could be considered "kinky" by someone else. Regardless of what you call your interests, tapping into erotic energy is potent for transformation, and not just sexually.

Some folks who engage in BDSM activities don't become sexually aroused from it because that's not the goal. Instead, they seek the feelings or experiences they might not have in other areas of life, such as feelings of power (domination) or the release of responsibility (submission or restraint).

As a CEO and business owner, I must make decisions all day, months on end, about how to solve problems, delegate tasks, and deal with difficult situations. To say it's a lot of responsibility is an understatement. When I finish my day, the last thing I want to do is decide what to eat or deal with my chores. However, stepping into a "submissive role" in the evening with my husband is liberating. It helps me achieve important goals while feeling cared for by someone else.

For instance, one evening, I came out of my office from working with clients via video conferencing, and it was a day of heavy topics. All I wanted to do was flop on the couch and do nothing, but I'd bitch at myself the next day if I left my chores for another time. Since my husband and I are in an agreed-upon power dynamic, he took a dominant role by telling me (in his very sexy Slovak accent), "I've ordered your favorite Mexican dish for delivery. I know you'll feel better about yourself if you fold your clothes and straighten up your office for tomorrow. If you do that while waiting for the food to arrive, I'll reward you by drawing a hot bath after dinner."

I mean, come on! Drool, right?

That event had nothing to do with sex and everything to do with the energy of relinquishing control while still being empowered through personal growth and valuable belief systems.

Did that experience eventually lead to sex? Absolutely! But not that night. I was too drained and pleasantly relaxed after my bath. However, since I have long on-ramps and high Erotic Exploration and Energetic Connection totals, the erotic energy from being taken care of and adored in that interaction fueled my arousal system for *days.*

Eroticizing chores and emotional needs are ways to connect with vitalizing (sometimes arousing) energy even around the mundane—we call it "Erotic Management."

Furthermore, erotic energy conceptualized through the Arousal Architecture® can provide space for folks to explore this vitality who are asexual or don't want intimacy reduced to sex or sexuality, as the author of *Asexual Erotics* explains.[4]

That's the power of understanding everything in this book and tapping into the Arousal Architecture® for your arousal potential and a more satisfying sex life. When you consider practices that can integrate aspects of the Arousal Architecture® dimensions into your daily life or relationship, it transcends typical sex acts into compelling experiences that ignite passion and deepen connection. Erotic energy can be the solution for captivating lives most people ache for.

Even if you don't identify strongly as a "sexual person," the Erotic Exploration dimension can offer opportunities to expand passionate energy within yourself. For instance, it can also refer to feeling an energetic pull toward someone or something that you wouldn't describe as sexual. You feel an attraction, but it's not sexually arousing.

The Erotic Exploration dimension concentrates on seeking and expanding your comfort zone and developing passionate pleasure (sexual or otherwise). In other Arousal Architecture® dimensions, the aim is to focus on seeking joy or pleasant sensations that arise. Regarding the Erotic Exploration dimension, the objective is to seek expansive, heated indulgence or excitement.

Furthermore, this dimension includes the power of play. As adults, we need to remember how crucial unstructured leisure time is. Typically, most folks spend it on passive entertainment, such as scrolling on social media or watching television. To flourish in life, reduce anxiety and depression, and increase the potential for arousal, we also need to create active leisure time to stimulate the parts of our brains and bodies that inspire connection, creativity, and a sense of flourishing. I loved learning acroyoga because it was the first time in my adult life that I had a consistent time set aside for playfulness. It was one of the reasons acro was profoundly healing. Not only was it pleasurable, but I could also focus on the fun experience without a goal or pressure.

A motto I love using is "Seek Pleasure." It's a reminder to constantly search for exciting, inspiring, and abundant experiences in everyday life. Connecting to my creative fire like this when I was dealing with sexual pain was one of the contributing factors that helped me through that emotionally painful time of life. I was able to redirect the energy I would typically use in sexual experiences to other endeavors that felt similarly fulfilling or vitalizing.

The concept of "pleasure" can be painful for folks when it's associated with sex and arousal because they feel pressure to experience it or disappointment that they don't have the kind of pleasure they desire. I offer eroticism as an expanded concept of pleasure to help folks reclaim it and seek similar types of fiery pleasure typically restricted to sex. Accessing pleasure in this new perspective can elicit empowerment and offer more opportunities for passion than you might have realized is possible. In the best-case scenario, by focusing on indulgent pleasure without the expectation of sexual arousal, you can create pathways to more easily access sexual arousal in time (if that's something you desire).

Overall, the on-ramps for the Erotic Exploration dimension are experiences that help you expand the edges of your comfort zone, engage in playful and empowering activities, or facilitate passionate and edgy sensual contexts. Off-ramps typically related to this dimension might be thoughts, ideas, or behaviors that feel disempowering, stifling, or routine.

How Does Trauma Relate to the Erotic Exploration Dimension?

Some questions in the Arousal Architecture® assess for adverse or traumatic past experiences because those can be barriers to arousal and sexual satisfaction even if they aren't related to sex or sexual trauma. Folks often feel shame or guilt that those experiences impact their sex lives. Since power is a core concept in the Erotic Exploration dimension and is practically an antidote to shame, interventions inspired by this dimension can help someone with past trauma reclaim power.

Working with trauma through the lens of erotic energy (either sexual energy or otherwise) is a potent process, and I recommend doing this with someone specialized. Usually, a licensed professional, such as a somatically focused trauma therapist or trauma-informed sex therapist, is my standard choice. However, some clients have found a lot of healing through working with professional Dominants at local dungeons. If you're interested in that route, get personal references or at least vet the potential professional however possible. If you're in Los Angeles or Portland, I can probably offer a few recommendations; please feel free to reach out!

Healing with a trusted professional can be essential in gaining power back over sexuality and arousal if you have unresolved trauma. You can also find potent ways to support your empowerment journey using exercises from this dimension.

Erotic Exploration Dimension Examples

Leaning into the Erotic Exploration dimension can feel unnerving, especially if you've never realized what eroticism can be. I can promise that no matter your score, there's something in this dimension for you; it just takes a little discovery and an open mind.

For example, James (he/him) enjoyed being playful and roughhousing with friends and siblings growing up, so we identified that intense sensuality could be an erotic energy to explore with a partner. However, James knew he didn't like the idea of getting spanked, so in the Arousal Architecture® workshop, I helped him identify the exciting ideas (wrestling, hair pulling, and firm grabbing) to request from partners while listing "spanking" under his "hard limits."

Another example comes from Bella (she/her), whose partner wanted to explore more erotic areas of their sexuality. However, she felt overwhelmed by her assumptions about what this meant. After talking with him, she realized his requests weren't the images of dark dungeons or latex suits she presumed. Mainly, he wanted novel experiences with their sex lives. Still, she wasn't sure how to comfortably do that because she wasn't familiar with creative or kinky sexuality. I suggested she start with an aspect of "sensory deprivation," such as wearing an eye mask during sexual play or asking him to hold her hands behind her back or over her head to restrict some of her movements. These options felt accessible to her and easy to pivot from in case she decided she didn't like playing with them.

The following are some examples of experiences or contexts in the Erotic Exploration dimension. I have provided more examples than the other dimensions to demonstrate how expansive this dimension can be.

- Engaging in playful or teasing banter (during sexual play or not).
- Creating something you're passionate about.
- Embracing fetishes (getting turned on by something that isn't typically sexual but is used for sexual arousal).
- Finding yourself in a "non-sexual" flow state.
- Touching parts of the body while intentionally avoiding genitals in a teasing way with yourself or a partner.

- Getting sexually creative, such as trying new sexual positions, role play, or using food erotically.
- Enjoying porn, erotica, or romance novels with edgy or kinky sex scenes.
- Experiencing attraction toward something where you anticipate desire even if you don't define it as sexual.
- Engaging in fantasy outside of sexual or erotic experiences such as enjoying sci-fi or fantasy movies or novels, dressing up in cosplay, or playing fantasy-inspired board games.

What Your Dimension Total Reveals About Your Arousal Language

Total = 6+

If you have a high level in the Erotic Exploration dimension, it could mean that sexual play and arousal feel more intense if you lovingly push against the edge of your comfort and expand the boundaries of pleasure. You enjoy savoring contexts and experiences that capture the essence of sexuality, especially if it's outside of the mainstream. Your arousal or interest in sex is likely enhanced by using your imagination and bringing sexual play beyond what society tells us is "normal." It means that you probably have the capacity (or desire) to utilize many ways to bring aliveness to sexual play and arousal possibilities.

If you have sexual challenges and a high total, it could imply that your sexual, erotic, or relational needs are not being met. Further, it might reveal a desire to explore more edgy experiences but feeling ashamed or embarrassed by those interests.

Many couples in sex therapy often have challenges around unspoken power dynamics within the relationship, and this could occur if one or more partners desire power dynamics but don't openly discuss how to navigate them.

Another aspect of the Erotic Exploration dimension that could be lacking for you is the experience of vitality or passionate energy in your life, sexually or overall.

Total = 0–5

Let's say you have a low total in the Erotic Exploration dimension. In that case, it doesn't mean anything less exciting about you and your needs, nor does it mean you don't want to push up against the "norm." It simply tells us that you don't need erotic energy to become aroused, or it is less influential to you. A low number in the Erotic Exploration dimension indicates you have other helpful dimensions to explore and focus on. However, as a sex therapist, I always believe we have room to grow, so if you want to learn how to make sex and arousal something that transcends to higher arousal potential, I'm here for it!

Sexual challenges and a low total could reflect similar indications as with a high total concerning difficulties connecting with a sense of vital or sensual energy or a willingness to push on the edges of your comfort zone (even gently). These explorative experiences could create opportunities for expanding growth or interests. You might also relate to feelings of depression, lack of passion or depth in your life, or rigidity. If you choose to explore, a little adventure could help spark a fire if done gradually and intentionally.

Suggestions and Interventions for Erotic Exploration Dimension

Exercises for Optimizing Your Erotic Exploration Dimension

- Use the Cognitive and Somatic Reframe exercise from Chapter 7 to rewrite your sexual narrative with an updated understanding of your sexual or erotic interests.

- Expand on your on- and off-ramps from Chapter 7 with an erotic perspective.
- Spend time cultivating experiences and thoughts that feel indulgent, passionate, and pleasant without a focus or expectation on sexual arousal.
- Enhance your erotic repertoire or find new interests by attending a workshop for new sexual skills, role play, or BDSM.

Want to Increase or Reduce Your Dimension Total?

Similar to the other dimensions, consider the influence the Erotic Exploration dimension has and determine if you might feel better served by improving the impact of the other dimensions before trying to decrease this one. Whether you want to reduce or increase the influential effect of the Erotic Exploration dimension, the following interventions can provide possibilities for enhancing your sexual self in ways that feel more authentic and pleasurable.

- Revisit and expand the Sexual Pleasure Paradigm Shift from Chapter 6 to consider new aspects to add to it with flavors of eroticism. Then, add them to your Sexual Menu from Chapter 9.
- Make time for playfulness (not necessarily sexually).
- Seek pleasure in areas of your life that feel innovative, enticing, or luxurious—however you define it.
- Explore a kinky or BDSM version of the "Yes, No, Maybe" List to get ideas (you'll find some in Part 4, but there are plenty of expanded versions you can find online).
- Consider areas of your life that feel playful and try to find ways to eroticize them.

Exercises

Quick Win!

Identify your top three to five ideal Erotic Exploration contexts or experiences and explore the meaning.

Going Deeper

For a refresher on the detailed instructions, refer to the end of Chapter 8.

Reflect on your responses to the questions you most responded to when you answered. Then, examine *why* you answered the way you did or interview yourself with the relevant questions from the "5W and H" journalism technique ("Who?" "What?" "Why?" etc.).

14

Your Arousal Design and Exploration

Now that you have learned about the Arousal Architecture® and its dimensions, let's look at practical applications of using your newfound information about yourself from this process.

If you only used the *Quick Win!* exercise prompts to identify your top items in each dimension, you likely have a list of fifteen to twenty-five thoughts, behaviors, or contexts that create your Arousal Architecture® design.

Using these, you can discover authentic and fulfilling pathways to arousal. Some of them might not be explicitly sexual. Instead, they are your motivators that can inspire you to engage in sexual play. They also might be options to increase nervous system regulation or overall quality of life.

Some of the items in your design could be directly related to the kind of sexual play you want or enjoy. These are experiences or contexts that keep you on the Sexy Time Track and are a part of your sexual self and arousal language.

Knowing your Arousal Architecture® design and how you want aspects of your design in your life creates more self-awareness. It also enables you to access concrete language to share with your partner(s) so they can help create a satisfying and pleasure-filled sexual experience with you. Furthermore, you can refer to your Arousal Architecture® design when you need a little reminder of what works for you, or you're drawing blanks on your creative possibilities.

When we're used to the same sexual routines and patterns, it can be difficult to remember new experiences you want to have instead.

There's nothing wrong with referring to your design (or your partner's) as regularly as you need. It's not less sexy or romantic. In fact, your intentional efforts to invest in cultivating an authentic and pleasure-focused sex life are incredibly hot.

The following are examples of what the Arousal Architecture® designs (or lists) might look like for Partners A and B, as illustrated in Figures 14.1 and 14.2, respectively, whose results you saw in Chapter 8. As a reminder, these were their totals:

Partner A

- Sexual Stimulation: 3
- Embodied Experience: 8
- Mental Headspace: 6
- Energetic Connection: 9
- Erotic Exploration: 3

Partner B

- Sexual Stimulation: 9
- Embodied Experience: 2
- Mental Headspace: 3
- Energetic Connection: 7
- Erotic Exploration: 8

My Faves Related to Sexual Stimulation:

1. Make out sessions.
2. Oral sex.
3. Plenty of sensual touching before my genitals are touched.

My Faves Related to Embodied Experience:

1. When the room has soft lighting and a comfortable temperature.
2. Spending time snuggling with my partner naked or in underwear.
3. A regular exercise routine.
4. Using my senses to ground myself in the present moment, especially during sex.

My Faves Related to Mental Headspace:

1. Mindful walking meditation.
2. Dirty talk during sexual play (or throughout the day sexting).
3. Words of admiration throughout the day.
4. Finishing my to-do list.

My Faves Related to Energetic Connection:

1. Having deep and connected conversations with my partner about our day.
2. Words of adoration, such as hearing my partner loves me when we're having sex.
3. When my partner looks at me with desire and love.

My Faves Related to Erotic Exploration:

1. Sexual play on vacation, especially in fancy hotels we've never visited before.
2. Hearing about my partner's fantasies that involve me.
3. When my partner takes control in sex or fun and playful activities.

FIGURE 14.1 *The Arousal Architecture® Top Faves journal entry for Partner A.*

Hopefully, with these examples and your explorations, you'll feel a lot more confident in rewriting your sexual narratives with your tangible and concrete ideas for reclaiming authentic pleasure and sexual power.

The *Going Deeper* exercises might have helped you expand your understanding of your sexual self and wellness needs. You can continue

My Faves Related to Sexual Stimulation:

> 1. Penetrative sex (any kind).
> 2. Seeing my partner naked, especially right after a shower.
> 3. When my partner tells me they want sex.
> 4. Knowing we're going to have sex later in the day or evening.
> 5. Watching my partner in pleasure.

My Faves Related to Embodied Experience:

> 1. Feeling fit in my body.
> 2. Holding my partner close to me in the morning as we wake up.

My Faves Related to Mental Headspace:

> 1. Dirty talk throughout the day and during sex.
> 2. Hearing my partner express pleasure because of me.

My Faves Related to Energetic Connection:

> 1. Knowing and experiencing my partner's love and commitment to me.
> 2. Being told how grateful my partner feels for our relationship.
> 3. Seeing the desire in my partner's eyes for me.
> 4. Taking my partner out on romantic dates and seeing their joy.

My Faves Related to Erotic Exploration:

> 1. Feeling in control of sexual play with my partner.
> 2. Playfully teasing my partner or engaging in banter together.
> 3. Trying new positions, implements, or using toys in our sexual play.
> 4. Role play, such as attending events or parties, dressing up in cocktail attire, and pretending we've just met at the bar.

FIGURE 14.2 *The Arousal Architecture® Top Faves journal entry for Partner B.*

to explore in similar ways over time, grow, and learn about yourself constantly.

With time, this curiosity style can become a natural part of your self-awareness development, leading to a more robust sense of self.

Question from the Sexual Stimulation Dimension:

> "Reaching orgasm is not usually a challenge for me."

Response Exploration:

> It's not usually an issue when I'm on my own with a vibrator. It's usually much easier before I go to sleep and I prefer to have the covers over most of my body. I have a difficult time without a vibrator or with a partner.

Insights + Interventions to Optimize or Adjust this Dimension

> I know orgasm is possible, but I have some barriers in certain situations that I would like to address. Communicating about my on- and off-ramps with my partner will be helpful. I can also use the vibrator with my partner.

On-Ramps Related to Sexual Stimulation Dimension:

> - Knowing my partner is eager to use lube.
> - Agreeing there's no expectation for orgasm or penetration.
> - Focusing on pleasure in whatever way feels right for me at the moment.

Off-Ramps Related to Sexual Stimulation Dimension:

> - Chest or genitals being touched when I'm not aroused or prepared for it.
> - Overtly sexual comments or activities without warm-up with other types of touch, conversation, or experiences.

FIGURE 14.3 *Arousal, Answered™ Workbook exploration entry example.*

Now, suppose you have sexual challenges, and the Arousal Architecture® design sheds some light on areas you're struggling with. In that case, you can use the information you learned by identifying parts of your sexual self that you would like to shift—using your Arousal Architecture® design along with the *Going Deeper* exercise and the following prompts to uncover possibilities to move forward.

- What did you uncover that you would like to shift or think could keep you from optimizing each dimension?

- What interventions in the dimension resonated with you? If none, what do you need help with?

- What are your on- and off-ramps related to your challenges, and how can they support you in overcoming them?

Figure 14.3 gives an example of Partner A using the *Arousal, Answered® Workbook*.

Partner A realized that exploring her response to the Arousal Architecture® question allowed her to target something she had been struggling with but didn't know how to tackle. She thought this was how it would be and held a lot of shame around it, thinking something was wrong with her. However, concrete steps and a road map for how to overcome this obstacle helped her feel more empowered and eventually experience orgasm with a partner.

The Arousal Architecture® is your road map for optimizing sexual wellness. It's your guide, providing you with concrete ideas to support rewriting your sexual narrative and embracing your authentic sexual self.

Now, it's your turn! Use the prompts here or check out my website for the *Arousal, Answered® Workbook*.

PART 4

IMPLEMENTATION AND APPLICATION

Supported by a solid foundation of sexual science and mind-body wellness, you are now poised to transform your sexual narrative. Utilizing the principles of neuroscience, somatics, and mindset, you have the tools to cultivate an optimal environment for your mind, body, and energy to harness the power of the Arousal Architecture®.

The Arousal Architecture® assessment results have provided you with a road map to embrace your authentic sexual self, enhancing your arousal and pleasure potential.

The following chapters will help you integrate the information into your routines and everyday circumstances. Furthermore, you'll learn communication strategies that make it easier to overcome hurdles with partners and inspire confidence, knowing you can communicate about what you want and need. I've introduced some of my favorite interventions and exercises for continued support as you live your new sexual narrative.

Additionally, you'll learn foundational skills to navigate and communicate with healthcare providers if you have sexual challenges that you wish to seek medical support for in case you've been dealing with issues for over six months. Getting a medical rule out is always helpful so you know what to focus on in your healing journey. It's surprising to know how many medications have sexual side effects that doctors don't mention. Being direct with your providers about your challenges can significantly affect your treatment plan and quality of life.

15

How to Use Your New Transformational System in Daily Life

All the content you've digested can be life-changing if you actively integrate it into your life. Use what you've learned from the Arousal Architecture® results to prioritize experiences or contexts that help you access sexual arousal, even if that means you prefer to focus on nervous system regulation or engage in self-care activities. Essentially, with the Arousal Architecture® design, you can build the on-ramps and remove the potential off-ramps by doing more of what you or your partner enjoys and avoiding situations that get you off track. You now have concrete action items and a road map, so you don't have to guess what works and what doesn't.

Remember, the *Quick Win!* exercises are perfectly adequate interventions to add to your regular routines if you ever feel overwhelmed trying to do everything. Using the Arousal Architecture® design can help you narrow down the exercises to focus on. For instance, if you have high totals in the Mental Headspace and Embodied Experience dimensions, lean more toward including mindfulness and somatic exercises in your daily routine or sexual play.

I use this process with private clients to create their Sexual Wellness Plans. Now, you have the tools to create your own by identifying your needs, the suggested interventions you resonated with, and what your partner needs and wants (if you have a partner you wish to do this with). For instance, plan your days and weeks integrating sexual wellness activities or contexts as you would meal planning.

Improving your arousal, pleasure, and sex life takes effort. It doesn't just transform because you've increased your sexual health knowledge or unlocked new understandings about yourself (or a partner). Being intentional about creating opportunities for sexual or romantic experiences is a fantastic way to keep passion and arousal as consistent parts of your life. You might experience ebbs and flows, so take comfort in knowing your sexual flow will eventually come back when you continue to practice self-care, mental and physical wellness, and relational engagement.

You now have the most foundational content and education I've seen my clients need to access authentic arousal and satisfying sex lives. Go forth and seek pleasure!

How to Continue Optimizing Self-Love and Sexy Times

The following content comprises supplemental exercises and interventions I've used with clients and students over the past two decades. I'm thrilled to share them with you. Some are introductory or basic outlines since I can't get as detailed as in private sessions or programs. However, they're still effective and will facilitate momentum in rewriting your sexual narrative regardless. I have included them here because they can be applied to multiple dimensions and used in various ways—whether you're dating yourself or someone else.

I aim to provide options for you to experience change without feeling like a burden or overwhelming your schedule. These are simply suggestions, so feel free to do only some or all! If you're not ready to incorporate them now, that's okay—they'll be here for you when and if you want to use them.

Pleasure-Bombing

When sexual arousal and experiences have been fraught with tension or disappointment, it can feel hard to get the engine running again. Sometimes, all that's needed is a little fuel and constant exposure to pleasurable contexts (in ways that work for you).

I'll often recommend clients to get exposure through reading saucy romance novels, listening to audio erotica, or watching body-positive and ethical porn. However, it's crucial to remove expectations to do anything besides the exposure—meaning, don't add pressure to feel aroused or engaged in sexual play. The more you create sexual contexts around you without tension, the easier it will be to jump-start your arousal system when you're ready.

This suggestion isn't a surefire way to do this, and it might not be for everyone. Sometimes, I need to workshop this with clients to find something that does work for them. So, if you like the idea of doing this but it feels clumsy, awkward, or ineffective, you might need to give it some time or adjust when and what kinds of pleasure you're exposing yourself to. Use the Arousal Architecture® design to target the dimensions you have higher totals in and help you decide on the types of content you think will work best for you.

"Yes, No, Maybe" List

A "Yes, No, Maybe" List is a compilation of sensual, sexual, erotic, or kinky behaviors or contexts that you can indicate if each item is something you're interested in or not, and you can indicate a "maybe" if you're open to it but in certain situations.

"Yes, No, Maybe" List (+ Kinky Options)

ACTIVITY (ROLE)	YES	NO	MAYBE
Oral Sex (giving)	○	○	○
Oral Sex (receiving)	○	○	○
Using sex toys (alone)	○	○	○
Using sex toys (w/ others)	○	○	○
Dirty Talk (giving)	○	○	○
Dirty Talk (receiving)	○	○	○
Spanking (giving)	○	○	○
Spanking (receiving)	○	○	○
Using restraints in sex (giving)	○	○	○
Using restraints in sex (receiving)	○	○	○
Exhibitionism	○	○	○

FIGURE 15.1 *Yes, No, Maybe List (+ Kinky Options) exercise.*

It's a great way to get ideas for your Sexual Menu from Chapter 9 and an effective tool to communicate with a partner about shared interests and limitations you each have.

You can create your own, search for one online, or check out Chapter 19 for ones I've enjoyed. Figure 15.1 gives an example of how one might look with some kinky options.

Write a Love Letter

To Yourself

Write a letter to yourself. It can be short or long. Don't edit yourself or judge the words that flow through your mind to your hands as you write them. After a few months, revisit the letter and notice if anything has changed.

If you are (or start) dating another person, notice if your partner has said these things about or to you. It's amazing what happens when we put our desires down in something concrete—we can often create the life we want. It's pretty magical!

Here are some suggestions for this letter:

- Think of all the ways you love yourself and let yourself know.
- Tell yourself the things you would love to hear from a partner.
- Explain the aspects of yourself you admire.
- Validate the experiences you've had and need love around.
- Recognize the accomplishments you've had and the difficulties you've faced.
- Celebrate overcoming obstacles and personal growth you've navigated.
- Take responsibility for neglecting any of your needs and explain how you will prevent them in the future.
- Commit to values and ways you would like to uplevel your life.

To a Partner

Use the same questions above to write a letter to a partner. You might not even wish to share it with them, but you can, of course, if you want! If your partner has a high Embodied Connection total, they would probably love reading it.

Ask a Partner to Write One to You

Even if you don't have a high total in the Embodied Connection dimension, you might love this exercise anyway! It's always wonderful to hear the things that our partners think of us but might not say as often as we would like to hear.

Provide your partner with the prompts above and add or remove anything you'd like. Change "yourself" to "your partner" and other alterations, as applicable.

How to Flirt and Talk Dirty

I've grouped these two together because they are similar—one is just "naughtier." The suggestions that follow skim the surface because there is so much I could include, but it could fill a whole other book!

Overall, you'll enjoy flirting or talking dirty more when you reflect that you're listening to what matters to this person.

Flirting isn't just for single folks! If you've learned about your partner's Arousal Architecture® design, you already have insight on how to light their fire. You can use items from their Arousal Architecture® or read between the lines about what excites them.

Use a dimension's context to comment on something about them. For example, suppose they have a high total in Mental Headspace and share they're proud of a recent accomplishment. In that case, you might say, "Wow, smart, funny, and attractive . . . how did I get so lucky?"

When flirting with a stranger, engage in Active Listening (when you hear what they say and are attuned to their thoughts and feelings). Use the information you gather about them in conversation or observations to flirt.

Flirting should be fun and playful, without an ulterior motive. Enjoy the interaction itself, not just the outcome. Do it for novelty and to make a moment more interesting than the humdrum of daily life. That can help reduce the pressure on it for you.

Flirting can be verbal or physical (where appropriate), such as a slight touch that makes you wonder if they meant to do it or not. The thought that they intentionally meant to touch you could be hot and exciting.

Tips for Flirting

- Conversation tips:
    - Make conversations fun and humorous.
    - Compliment non-appearance aspects if you're flirting with a stranger. Follow up with questions related to the compliment.
    - Reflect observations positively or playfully.
    - Be creative and genuine with compliments. Avoid generic phrases like "you're so hot."

- Read the room. Flirt only when the energy is right and welcomed. Avoid serious or negative moments.
- Use light teasing and inside jokes to create a playful connection. Ensure it's good-natured and not hurtful. Two-way teasing (or banter) can be thrilling.
- Be suggestive without being explicit. Keep the flirting subtle and intriguing.

Tips for Talking Dirty

Start with something that feels accessible to you. You can try it with sexting so you have time to think about what you want to say and room for retyping. Or, if you're in person, you could blindfold your partner so they can't see you when you feel like you're flubbing responses.

- Say what you're feeling or observing.
  - It can be super simple: "You really turn me on." "I love how your body feels on me." "I can't wait to be in (on) you."
- You can ask for or give feedback, which is two wins in one because you're communicating about wants and needs and making it hot!
  - Harder, softer, more, a little to the left.
  - The way you're touching me is so hot.
  - Do you like how I do that to you?
  - Does that feel good when I do [that thing] to you?

Most importantly, know that when you're attempting to increase flirting or dirty talk, you'll likely feel uncertain or even awkward. Refer to the Mindset suggestions at the beginning of the book and gain confidence by practicing and being compassionate with yourself!

How to Navigate Sexual Challenges with Healthcare Providers

While this might not be an everyday scenario, getting a medical rule out is beneficial if you've been dealing with challenges for over six months. Navigating sexual difficulties can be demanding, especially if you need to discuss them with healthcare providers who aren't specialized in sexual medicine. In that case, it will be helpful to know how to talk about these issues in a way that helps you feel empowered and confident with doctors.

Let's say you're going to see a gynecologist, urologist, or sex therapist. You've likely waited months to get the appointment, and you only have a short time with them. To make the most of the appointment, prepare by thinking about the points below or writing notes for yourself.

- For a few weeks before the appointment, use a Pain Diary or Symptom Tracker so you have reliable data to discuss your concerns.
  - Include when you notice the symptoms improving or worsening and other components that might influence your body or issues. If you experience pain or uncomfortable sensations, expand on the sensations as best as you can (e.g., burning, stinging, throbbing, deep, surface level).
  - Note the places on your body or genitals where you experience the pain or sensation. The Mirror Exercise from Chapter 6 is a helpful guide. Make sure to identify the exact places where you experience the discomfort.
- Create an organized plan and talking points.
  - Clarify what you need to know about your concern.

- Briefly provide a history. Bullet points and a timeline are constructive.
- Identify your presenting concern, symptoms, or diagnosis(ses).
• Take notes and ask for a straightforward treatment plan.

Healthcare providers love it when patients are organized and concise. But don't feel pressured to limit what you say or the help you need. A clear outline will help you feel more grounded and confident.

If you want a free download with a printable handout to fill in and take to your next appointment, you can get my Patient Empowerment Handout from my website: www.cassardcenter.com/freebies.

16

How to Talk About Sex More Effectively

Having all the sexual knowledge and incredible intimacy models in the world is pointless if you don't know how to effectively talk about what you want and need. Plus, if you're not able to give and receive feedback, assert boundaries, or understand your partner's needs without becoming defensive, blaming yourself, or shutting down, it will be more challenging to have the kind of sex life you want and deserve.

We're not taught how to talk about sex in healthy ways. Most of my programs, education, and therapy sessions are about effective communication because most people need to overhaul their communication strategies. The content that follows summarizes the most beneficial suggestions and steps to take so you can confidently apply what you've learned in the book to your dating situation, whatever it looks like. I didn't include basic communication tools that you can easily search for online (like using "I statements"), so if you don't know what those are, that's where Dr. Google can be a great resource!

Build Your Communication Toolbox

Knowing what you want to say and what your goal is before you talk with another person about sexual topics is essential. Often, partners complain that they don't feel heard or listened to. While a portion of that responsibility might rely on the other person, there are some aspects that you can prepare for to support healthy conversations.

Preface Conversations with a Request

Most people typically assume others know what we want from a conversation. However, this is a source of conflict for many people in relationships. You might engage in a conversation looking for empathy or compassion, but your partner may respond with problem-solving. I'm guilty of this on both sides!

Before conversing with someone, think about what you desire from them in their response.

Do you want to vent and receive compassion or empathy, or would you like them to help with problem-solving, or are you seeking their opinion?

Once you've identified it, preface the conversation with your preferences. A bonus is to ask if they are available for what you're looking for.

After a long day, I've asked my husband if he's available for me to rant and vent about my frustrating day. Sometimes, he says "no." I appreciate hearing it; otherwise, we would have had a frustrating conversation if he hadn't honored his boundaries and needs. In the past, I would have just dumped on him, and he would push through, being the supportive husband he is. However, because he was already tired, his responses were short or unengaged, and I could see his eyes glazing over. I would leave the conversation disconnected, and he would be even more drained.

When we started making requests and checking in with each other's availability, it became much easier for us to have authentic and engaged conversations while respecting our ability to protect our energy when necessary.

As I'll explain, providing an alternative when someone is unavailable is also beneficial for this process.

Levels of Communication

Sometimes, couples complain that one partner wants a deeper connection. The other partner doesn't fully understand what their partner means because they believe they've talked plenty. However, there are multiple layers to conversations about the same thing. Folks are surprised to learn there can be numerous ways to interpret and respond to the question, "How was your day?"

Consider these three layers of communication for that question:

1. *Superficial Level*: This is factually based information or a narration of the day's events.
   - "I met with my boss in the afternoon and then picked up the prescriptions after work."
2. *Emotional Level*: Expressing feelings or emotions about the day's event.
   - "I was stressed about the meeting with my boss and worried about the side effects of using this new medication."
3. *Meaning Level*: This is the more significant impact of the events and the meaning someone makes about them.
   - "I was stressed about the meeting with my boss because the company is downsizing, and so much feels uncertain. Then, when the pharmacist told me about the potential side effects of the medication, I reconsidered taking it. Now, I feel unclear about the next steps in managing my health, and I'm doubting my decisions around the treatment plan I discussed with the doctor."

Identify the level of communication you desire in advance and let the other person know. Also, check in with your energetic resources and determine what you're available for. You might be exhausted and only have the energy to support your partner for Level 1 or 2 conversations. If that's the case, let them know. Reassure them by offering another time you're available for Level

3 conversations. In the meantime, suggest something else that might help in a way you can, such as a hug or cuddle.

Provide Effective Feedback with a Compliment Sandwich

The Compliment Sandwich is a tool for saying "no" or "maybe" or for giving feedback to someone else.

For instance, let's say your partner indicates they want something sexual that you don't want. You can say "no" while staying connected by using this process:

1. Start with a positive or affirming statement.
   - "I love that you want to be close to me."
2. Give your feedback.
   - "I have more responsive desire, so when you ask me if I want sex tonight, I don't always know."
3. End with a positive or affirming statement.
   - "I want to be close to you and enjoy it when we cuddle and play with each other's hair. Doing that usually makes me want more with you, so can we start there?"

You can also shorten this when in the middle of sexual play, making it erotic with "dirty talk." For instance, imagine you need them to slow down how they're touching you. Telling them something like the phrase below keeps the sexy energy while still giving feedback about the kind of touch you prefer.

"I love feeling your touch on my body. Try a little slower."

Then, when they adjust in a way that feels better, respond with reassurance, such as, "Mmmm, yes, just like that."

It's okay if they don't adjust how you prefer on the first attempt. Continue to provide affirmative guidance and avoid words such as "not" or "don't." Instead, use phrases based on neutral descriptions such as "more," "less," "harder," or "softer."

How to Communicate When Dealing with Difficulties

Relationship challenges and sexual issues can complicate communication since they're emotionally weighted. It's even more challenging to implement change when you don't feel understood by your partner. Remember to use nervous system regulation tools such as mindfulness and somatic techniques before, during, and after difficult conversations. Doing so will make conversations more productive and rewire brain pathways for confidence and more connected intimacy (however you define it).

Communication Formula

I offer two-hour workshops on this intervention, but having the formula and trying it out on your own could be sufficient. If not, reach out, and I can help!

When you find yourself in a situation that requires a tough conversation about relationship issues, having a structured approach can be beneficial. The following is a "formula" that I've developed and refined over the past two decades, drawing from various models. Initially, it may feel rigid, but with practice, you'll find it seamlessly integrating into your conversations, leading to better outcomes!

1. When you said or did (state an observable behavior).
2. I felt (use a feeling or emotion word, not a belief).

3. I told myself this story: (explain how you interpreted it using "I statements" and the meaning you made of the situation).

4. What I need from you is (make a gentle request to help you feel better about the situation).

This formula can be incredibly helpful, but being aware of potential pitfalls is essential. For instance, in the second step, many people inadvertently introduce a belief about their partner by saying, "I feel like you don't love me." So, if you're using this formula and your second sentence starts with "I feel like . . ." pause and start again, focusing on the emotions you feel. This will ensure the formula's effectiveness in your conversations.

Another tip is about the gentle request in the fourth step. This part aims to ask for something that the other person can do proactively. When first practicing this process, some clients start with "I need you to know how I feel about this" if they feel uncertain about what to request.

How to Talk About Sexual Issues When Newly Dating

I love helping clients create "scripts" to discuss their needs in new dynamics or relationships based on their comfort levels and unique challenges. Below are common considerations to reflect on for deciding how and when to talk to a new partner about challenges you might experience in sexual situations.

- How long have you been dating? What do you want from the relationship?
- Do you think the relationship will last long enough that you'll confront the sexual situation regularly?
- Have they handled other vulnerable or sensitive topics well?
- What do you hope they will know after you've shared this with them?
- How do you hope they'll respond?

- Why is it essential for you to address this now? Is it beneficial to discuss it later (aside from being easier to avoid now)?
- What kind of support do you need to share this with them?

When you're clear about what you want and hope to achieve by sharing with them, provide some context about what you're sharing and how they can help support you.

If they are open and handle the conversation well, they will likely be able to handle other relationship road bumps well, too. However, if they don't, it's a good indicator that they might not have the tools to be an emotionally available or supportive partner.

AFTERWORD AND ADDITIONAL RESOURCES

Even though our journey together in this format is ending, I wanted to share some final thoughts with you.

While the goal of the book was to help you rewrite your sexual narrative, it was also to inspire you to stretch beyond your comfort zone. Pushing gently against your edges while using nervous system regulation skills expands the possibilities for pleasure and satisfaction. However, while you're expanding your comfort zone, it can feel challenging, awkward, and maybe even overwhelming. I recommend remembering your purpose for committing to change in those cases.

Consider reflecting on the ultimate reward of reshaping your relationship to sex, arousal, and pleasure: obtaining empowerment through taking control back from oppressive or sex-negative systems.

Remind yourself that all change can be difficult. Still, the benefits are potent, especially when you remember that a healthy and satisfying sex life highly correlates to relationship wellness and overall quality of life.

In case you need a motto or positive affirmation to support you through the transformation, you can use my most frequently recommended phrase: "I'm moving closer to rewiring my pleasure pathways and rewriting my sexual narrative."

Healing isn't a linear process. It's more like an upward spiral. As you go around the healing process in the spiral, you'll encounter similar challenges at the same vertical point in the upward progression. However, as you've accumulated a more profound understanding, you'll handle parallel challenges with a new perspective or problem-solving process you might not have discovered.

Hopefully, this helps you avoid self-judgment when some issues inevitably resurface. It's not that you haven't processed it properly or didn't learn from your past. Instead, you are now more experienced in confronting the potentially deeper levels of the issue that you might not have realized were there or prepared to address at the time.

If you still struggle after reading this book, my online courses, coaching programs, and therapy intensives can support your healing.

Even if you simply wish to optimize your sex life, arousal, and pleasure potential, I have programs and courses for that, too. Head over to www.cassardcenter.com/services to learn more.

Remember that several free resources are on the "freebies" page, or you can check out my YouTube channel for educational videos on sexual pain, anxiety, and wellness.

Further Resources

I've handpicked my favorite recommendations for you in addition to what you'll find on my website and in the references.

Please note that I've done the best I can with the information I had in these suggestions: an endorsement that follows does not support everything these resources or folks have done, nor does it say that I agree with everything they have ever said or done.

This list is not exhaustive; there might be many other fabulous folks and organizations. Please let me know if you think I should add someone to this list in future publications. I'm always happy to learn and grow.

I have partnered with some of the recommendations, and they have graciously provided discounts for my community that you can also access at www.cassardcenter.com/freebies.

Mindfulness Resources

- iChill app by the Trauma Resource Institute (www.traumaresourceinstitute.com/ichill)
- Headspace App
- Calm App

Neurodivergence

- ADDitude Magazine: An online resource for ADD, ADHD, and Autism. (www.additudemag.com)
- Jessica McCabe, creator of "How to ADHD," an online resource and YouTube channel for navigating neurodivergence. (www.howtoadhd.com)
- Dr. Neff: A psychologist creating resources for neurodivergent brains. (www.neurodivergentinsights.com, @neurodivergent_insights)

Painful Sex

- International Pelvic Pain Society (www.pelvicpain.org)
- *Tight-Lipped*: A grassroots movement by and for people with chronic vulvovaginal and pelvic pain. (www.tightlipped.org, @tightlippedorg)
- *The Pelvic People*, creator of devices to improve sexual pain, and The Pelvic Gym, online educational courses by clinicians and specialists. (www.thepelvicpeople.com)
- *GoLove CBD Intimate Serum* has a water-based lube-like consistency for moisturizing and relaxing pelvic muscles. (www.golovecbd.com)
- *VWell* creates pelvic health wands and dilators with medical-grade silicone. (www.vwell.com - use code KAYNA for a discount)

Sexual Health Wellness

- Asexuality and aromantics:
  - PFLAG: Non-profit organization with great LGBTQI+ and asexual or aromantic resources. (www.pflag.org/resource/ace-aro-resources, @pflag)
  - Asexual Agenda: A blog for asexual folks. (www.asexualagenda.wordpress.com)
- Fat-positive sexual healthcare with Sonalee Rashatwar, LCSW, MEd. (www.sonaleer.com, @thefatsextherapist)
- *Decolonizing Contraception* by the Restorative Justice Initiative (@reprojusticeinitiative)
- *Melt: Massage for Couples* has courses that make sensual massage accessible to anyone. (www.couplesmassagecourses.com)
- *Lorals* provides latex lingerie for fashion, playtime, comfort, and confidence. (www.mylorals.com)
- Online Educational Courses for sexual wellness skills:
  - OMGYes (www.omgyes.com)
  - Beducated (www.beducated.com)
- *Power to Decide*: High-quality, accurate information on sexual health and contraceptive methods so young people can make informed decisions. (www.powertodecide.org)
- *The Principles of Pleasure* on Netflix
- Sexological Bodyworkers (www.sexologicalbodyworkers.org/whatis)
- *SexPositive World Organization*: Worldwide and local communities, educational workshops, and events. (www.sexpositiveworld.org)
- Sex Surrogate Partners (www.surrogatetherapy.org)

- Yes, No, Maybe Lists:
  - By A.E. Osworth: https://www.autostraddle.com/you-need-help-here-is-a-worksheet-to-help-you-talk-to-partners-about-sex-237385/
  - By Bex: https://www.bextalkssex.com/yes-no-maybe/

AAPI Resources

- *AAPI Women Lead*: Resources for AAPI women, including those affected by sexual violence. (www.imreadymovement.org, @aapiwomenlead)
- *API Queer Women and Transgender Community* (APIQWTC): Provides opportunities for Asian & Pacific Islander queer women and transgender people to socialize, network, build community, engage in inter-generational organizing, and increase community visibility. (www.apiqwtc.org, @apiqwtc)
- *It Gets Better*: Resources for AAPI LGBTQ+ folks. (www.itgetsbetter.org, @itgetsbetter)
- *National Asian Pacific American Women's Foundation*: Organization aiming to build the power, influence, and autonomy of AAPI women and girls. (www.napawf.org, @napawf)

Black and African American Educators, Researchers, and Therapists and Sexual Wellness Resources for Black and African American Folks

- *Afrosexology*: Pleasure-based sex education platform for Black folks. (afrosexology.com, @afrosexology)
- *Black Female Therapists Directory* (@blackfemaletherapists)

- *Black Girls' Guide to Surviving Menopause* (@blackgirlsguidetomenopause)
- "Black Lives Matter Meditations" (not affiliated with the Black Lives Matter organization) by Dr. Candace Nicole Hargon (@dr.candicenicole)
- *Black Women's Pleasure Mapping* and #hotgirlscience by Dr. Shemeka Thorpe (@drshemeka), Dr. Jardin Dogan-Dixon (@blkfolxtherapy), Dr. Ashley Townes (@dr.ashleytownes), and Natalie Malone (@futuredr.nat)
- *Hoodrat to Headwrap*: A Decolonized Podcast by Erika Hart (@iharterika) and Ebony Donnley
- *Kimbritive* by Kimberly Huggins and Brittany Brathwaite (@kimbritive)
- *Triple Cripples*: Highlighting the lives and sexual stories of Black disabled women and non-binary people. (@triplecripples)

Faith-Based and Sex Positive Counseling and Education

- Rev. Beverly Dale (www.incarnationinstitute.org/videos)
- Rev. Dr. Lacette Cross (www.revdrl.com)
- Natasha Helfer (www.natashahelfer.com)

Latin and Latina/x Resources

- *Latino Network*: Their Sexuality Education program strives to remove the stigma associated with teen pregnancy, STIs, and gender and sexual orientation and increase conversations around health and sexuality. (www.latnet.org/sexuality-education, @latinonetwork)
- *National Latina Institute for Reproductive Justice*: Amplifies Latina/x voices to transform the systems and narratives to reclaim their bodies and lives. (www.latinainstitute.org, @latinainstitute)

Native American and Indigenous Peoples Resources

- *Native Youth Sexual Health Network*: Native and two-spirit mental health peer-support. (https://www.nativeyouthsexualhealth.com/peersupportmanual, @nyshn)

- *We R Native*: Resources for native youth, by native youth. (https://www.wernative.org/my-relationships/sexual-health, @wernative)

Somatic Therapies and Resources

- Sensorimotor Psychotherapy (www.sensorimotorpsychotherapy.org)
- Somatic Experiencing (www.traumahealing.org)
- Somatic Attachment Healing (www.theembodylab.com)
- Somatic Abolition (www.resmaa.com/movement)

Suicide Prevention Support

- Text "HOME" to 741-741 for the *Crisis Text Line* (24/7)
- Call 9-8-8 regarding depression or suicidal ideation. They offer dedicated BIPOC resources. (www.988lifeline.org, 24/7)
- *Trevor Project*: Support for LGBTQ young adults, 1-866-488-7386 (24/7)

ACKNOWLEDGMENTS

To all the people who helped me on my journey, I am eternally grateful.

The most profound expression of gratitude is to my clients. No words can express the privilege and honor it has been to be invited into your lives during vulnerable and critical times. Your stories and trust have helped me become the clinician I am today. Without you, this book would not be possible.

I owe a debt of gratitude to those who paved the way for me to share this content. This experience humbles me, and I genuinely believe I am standing on the shoulders of giants. My supervisors, mentors, and colleagues have been indispensable as I've stepped into my role as a clinician and author.

To everyone who engaged with the beta version of the Arousal Architecture® and provided invaluable feedback—you helped it evolve into what it is today.

To the superb topic experts, clinicians, and dear friends who reviewed, workshopped, and provided feedback and corrections, your contributions have enhanced the credibility and impact of this model and book. Thank you, Chimine Arfuso, PhD, Jennifer Burton, MFT, Jess Caming, Katrina Chersicla, Casie Danenhauer, DPT, Lark Dearborne, Greg Devore, PhD, Jack Ferry, Elle Freely, LCSW, Moushumi Ghose, MFT, Nicoletta Heidegger, LMFT, Ashley Manta, ABS, Jennifer Meyer, LPC, LMFT, Taylor Olandt, Stephanie Prendergast, MP, Tabatha Snyder, PharmD, MBA, Sarah Turner, and Kathy and Ozan Varol.

To my dearest friends who checked in and have been constant cheerleaders throughout the years and during the development of the Arousal Architecture® and this book, your support has meant the world to me.

Waylon Baumgardner, a childhood friend, product designer, and developer, thank you for bringing the online version of the Arousal Architecture® assessment to the masses.

Misha Pimas, thank you for the beautiful body artwork that graces these pages.

To my parents, without their lifelong love and support, I might not have dreamed of accomplishing what I have. My mom was my ride-or-die researcher and writing assistant, constantly impressing me with her ability to learn new things. Your dedication and love kept me going when I wanted to give up. My dad cheered me on and reminded me he was proud no matter what came of this endeavor.

Ján, my devoted husband, ensured I ate, showered, and remained (mostly) sane during the late nights, long writing-filled weekends, sporadic meltdowns, and self-doubt spirals. I was practically non-existent during this paramount moment of my life, but you kept me afloat. Your tech support for the online Arousal Architecture® assessment was also a gift from the stars when I wanted to pull my hair out, as I know you did, too. I love you more than words can express.

The team at Sex, Answered kept the company going when I needed to be absent while writing. You essentially helped keep food on my table.

To my many therapists, especially Heather, who helped me transform and remember the purpose of writing this book: to have fun and hopefully change some lives, even if only a handful. Writing this book has healed so much trauma (and possibly activated a fair share more for me to bravely work through).

Finally, my devout, soulful gratitude to Bridgid, Selene, Hekate, and Lilith, who believed in me and inspired my magick.

With love, gratitude, and a deep belief in the power of pleasure.

NOTES

Introduction

1   Anna Kessler et al., "The Global Prevalence of Erectile Dysfunction: A Review," *BJU International* 124, no. 4 (2019): 587–99; Raymond C. Rosen, "Prevalence and Risk Factors of Sexual Dysfunction in Men and Women," *Current Psychiatry Reports* 2, no. 3 (2000): 189–95; Marita P. McCabe et al., "Incidence and Prevalence of Sexual Dysfunction in Women and Men: A Consensus Statement from the Fourth International Consultation on Sexual Medicine 2015," *The Journal of Sexual Medicine* 13, no. 2 (2016): 144–52.

2   David A. Frederick et al., "What Keeps Passion Alive? Sexual Satisfaction is Associated with Sexual Communication, Mood Setting, Sexual Variety, Oral Sex, Orgasm, And Sex Frequency in a National US Study," *The Journal of Sex Research* 54, no. 2 (2017): 186–201.

3   Justin J. Lehmiller et al., "Less Sex, but More Sexual Diversity: Changes in Sexual Behavior during the COVID-19 Coronavirus Pandemic," *Leisure Sciences* 43 no. 1–2 (2020): 295–304, https://doi.org/10.1080/01490400.2020.1774016.

Part 1

1   Kathleen F. Flugel Colle et al., "Measurement of Quality of Life and Participant Experience with the Mindfulness-Based Stress Reduction Program," *Complementary Therapies in Clinical Practice* 16, no. 1 (2010): 36–40; Tantri Keerthi Dinesh et al., "Effectiveness of Mindfulness-Based Interventions on Well-Being and Work-Related Stress in the Financial Sector: A Systematic Review and Meta-Analysis Protocol," *Systematic Reviews* 11, no. 1 (2022); Bassam Khoury et al., "Mindfulness-Based Stress Reduction for Healthy Individuals: A Meta-Analysis," *Journal of Psychosomatic Research* 78, no. 6 (2015): 519–28.

Chapter 1

1 Vida Demarin and Sandra Morović, "Neuroplasticity," *Periodicum Biologorum* 116, no. 2 (2014): 209–11.

Chapter 2

1 Thomas Hanna, "The Field of Somatics," *Somatics* 1, no. 1 (1976): 30–4; Peter Levine, "Accumulated Stress, Reserve Capacity, and Disease" (PhD diss., University of California, Berkeley, 1976), 1–24.

2 Peter Levine, *Waking the Tiger: Healing Trauma: The Innate Capacity to Transform Overwhelming Experiences* (Berkeley: North Atlantic Books, 1997); Resmaa Menakem, *My Grandmother's Hands: Radicalized Trauma and the Pathway to Mending Our Hearts and Bodies* (Las Vegas: Central Recovery Press, 2017); Pat Ogden, Kekuni Minton, and Claire Pain, *Trauma and the Body: A Sensorimotor Approach to Psychotherapy* (New York: WW Norton & Company, 2006); Bessel A. Van der Kolk, *The Body Keeps the Score: Brain, Mind, and Body in the Healing of Trauma* (New York: Penguin Books, 2014).

3 Marie Kuhfuß et al., "Somatic Experiencing—Effectiveness and Key Factors of a Body-Oriented Trauma Therapy: A Scoping Literature Review," *European Journal of Psychotraumatology* 12, no. 1 (2021).

4 Frederick Matthias Alexander, *Man's Supreme Inheritance: Conscious Guidance and Control in Relation to Human Evolution in Civilization* (London: Methuen, 1918); Rodrigo Gozalo-Pascual et al., "Efficacy of the Myofascial Approach as a Manual Therapy Technique in Patients with Clinical Anxiety: A Randomized Controlled Clinical Trial," *Complementary Therapies in Clinical Practice* 51 (2023): 1–7; Ida P. Rolf, *Rolfing: Reestablishing the Natural Alignment and Structural Integration of the Human Body for Vitality and Well-Being* (New York: Simon & Schuster, 1989).

5 Elaine Miller-Karas, *Building Resilience to Trauma: The Trauma and Community Resiliency Models*, 2nd ed. (New York: Routledge, 2023).

Chapter 3

1 Bassam Khoury et al., "Mindfulness-Based Stress Reduction for Healthy Individuals: A Meta-analysis," *Journal of Psychosomatic Research* 78, no. 6 (2015): 519–28.

Chapter 4

1. Carol S. Dweck, *Mindset: The New Psychology of Success* (New York: Random House, 2006).

2. Allan Rechtschaffen, "Current Perspectives on the Function of Sleep," *Perspectives in Biology and Medicine* 41, no. 3 (1998): 359–90; "How Much Sleep Do I Need?," Sleep and Sleep Disorders, Centers for Disease Control and Prevention (CDC), last modified, September 14, 2022, https://www.cdc.gov/sleep/about_sleep/how_much_sleep.html.

3. Isyaku Salisu et al., "Perseverance of Effort and Consistency of Interest for Entrepreneurial Career Success: Does Resilience Matter?" *Journal of Entrepreneurship in Emerging Economies* 12, no. 2 (2020): 279–304.

4. Cristina M. Bostan, "The Role of Motivational Persistence and Resilience Over the Well-being Changes Registered in Time," *Symposion* 2, no. 2 (2015): 215–41.

5. Hanne Albert, "Psychosomatic Group Treatment Helps Women with Chronic Pelvic Pain," *Journal of Psychosomatic Obstetrics & Gynecology* 20, no. 4 (1999): 216–25; Sidney Cobb, "Social Support as a Moderator of Life Stress," *Psychosomatic Medicine* 38, no. 5 (1976): 300–14; Linda D. Kames et al., "Effectiveness of an Interdisciplinary Pain Management Program for the Treatment of Chronic Pelvic Pain," *Pain* 41, no. 1 (1990): 41–46; Hugh Worrall et al., "The Effectiveness of Support Groups: A Literature Review," *Mental Health and Social Inclusion* 22, no. 2 (2018): 85–93.

6. Ralf Schwarzer and Reinhard Fuchs, "Self-efficacy and Health Behaviours," in *Predicting Health Behavior*, ed. Mark Conner and Paul Norman (Buckingham: Open University Press, 1996), 163–96; Per-Anders Tengland, "Behavior Change or Empowerment: on the Ethics of Health-promotion Strategies," *Public Health Ethics* 5, no. 2 (2012): 140–53.

7. Jeff Olson, *The Slight Edge: Turning Simple Disciplines into Massive Success and Happiness* (Austin, TX: Greenleaf Book Group, 2013).

8. Phillippa Lally et al., "How Are Habits Formed: Modelling Habit Formation in the Real World," *European Journal of Social Psychology* 40, no. 6 (2010): 998–1009.

Part 2

1. Georgine Lamvu et al., "Chronic Pelvic Pain in Women: A Review," *Jama* 325, no. 23 (2021): 2381-91.; Jianzhong Zhang et al., "Chronic Prostatitis/Chronic Pelvic Pain

Syndrome: A Disease or Symptom? Current Perspectives on Diagnosis, Treatment, and Prognosis," *American Journal of Men's Health* 14, no. 1 (2020): 1557988320903200.

Chapter 5

1. Oakley Ray, "How the Mind Hurts and Heals the Body," *American Psychologist* 59, no. 1 (2004): 29.

2. "What is Stress?" Stress, World Health Organization, last modified February 21, 2023, https://www.who.int/news-room/questions-and-answers/item/stress.

3. Elaine Miller-Karas, *Building Resilience to Trauma: The Trauma and Community Resiliency Models*, 2nd ed. (New York: Routledge, 2023).

4. N. Prause, H. Cohen, and G. J. Siegl, "Effects of Adverse Childhood Experiences on Partnered Sexual Arousal Appear Context Dependent," *Sexual and Relationship Therapy* 38, no. 3 (2023): 479–94.

Chapter 6

1. Ellie Strachan and Betty Staples, "Masturbation," *Pediatrics in Review* 33, no. 4 (2012): 190–1.

2. Ashley Leonard, "An Investigation of Masturbation and Coping Style" (presentation, 38th Annual Western Pennsylvania Undergraduate Psychology Conference, Slippery Rock University, 2010); Roy J. Levin, "Sexual Activity, Health and Well-Being—The Beneficial Roles of Coitus and Masturbation," *Sexual and Relationship Therapy* 22, no. 1 (2007): 135–48; Aniruddha Das, "Masturbation in the United States," *Journal of Sex & Marital Therapy* 33, no. 4 (2007): 301–17.

3. Kathleen E. Merwin and Natalie O. Rosen, "Perceived Partner Responsiveness Moderates the Associations Between Sexual Talk and Sexual and Relationship Well-Being in Individuals in Long-Term Relationships," *The Journal of Sex Research* 3 (2019): 351–64.

4. Stephanie A. Prendergast and Elizabeth H. Rummer, *Pelvic Pain Explained: What Everyone Needs to Know* (Lanham, MD: Rowman & Littlefield Publishers, 2017).

5. "All Vulvas Are Beautiful," Netflix, last modified 2021, https://www.all-vulvas-are-beautiful.com/.

6   Federico Belladelli et al., "Worldwide Temporal Trends in Penile Length: A Systematic Review and Meta-Analysis," *The World Journal of Men's Health* 41, no. 4 (2023): 848–60.

7   Menelaos Apostolou, "Size Did Not Matter: An Evolutionary Account of the Variation in Penis Size and Size Anxiety," *Cogent Psychology* 3, no. 1 (2016): 1147933.

8   Maria Uloko, Erika P. Isabey, and Blair R. Peters "How Many Nerve Fibers Innervate the Human Glans Clitoris: A Histomorphometric Evaluation of the Dorsal Nerve of the Clitoris," *The Journal of Sexual Medicine* 20, no. 3 (2023): 247–52.

9   Debby Herbenick et al., "Women's Experiences with Genital Touching, Sexual Pleasure, and Orgasm: Results from a US Probability Sample of Women Ages 18 to 94," *Journal of Sex & Marital Therapy* 44, no. 2 (2018): 201–12.

10 Elizabeth A. Mahar, Laurie B. Mintz, and Brianna M. Akers, "Orgasm Equality: Scientific Findings and Societal Implications," *Current Sexual Health Reports* 12, no. 1 (2020): 24–32.

11 Adam Ostrzenski, "G-Spot Anatomy: A New Discovery," *The Journal of Sexual Medicine* 9, no. 5 (2012): 1355–9; Vincenzo Puppo and Ilan Gruenwald, "Does the G-Spot Exist? A Review of the Current Literature," *International Urogynecology Journal* 23 (2012): 1665–9.

12 Lauri Nummenmaa et al., "Topography of Human Erogenous Zones," *Archives of Sexual Behavior* 45 (2016): 1207–16.

13 Glenn N. Levine et al., "Sexual Activity and Cardiovascular Disease: A Scientific Statement from the American Heart Association," *Circulation* 125, no. 8 (2012): 1058–72.

14 Emily Nagoski, *Come as You Are: The Surprising New Science that Will Transform Your Sex Life* (New York: Simon & Schuster, 2015); Emily Nagoski, *Come Together: The Science (and Art!) of Creating Lasting Sexual Connections* (New York: Ballantine Books, 2024).

15 "Sexual Arousal," APA Psychology Dictionary, American Psychological Association (APA), last modified April 19, 2018, https://dictionary.apa.org/sexual-arousal.

16 Meredith L. Chivers et al., "Agreement of Self-reported and Genital Measures of Sexual Arousal in Men and Women: A Meta-analysis," *Archives of Sexual Behavior* 39, no. 1 (2010): 5–56.

17 Rosemary Basson, "The Female Sexual Response: A Different Model," *Journal of Sex & Marital Therapy* 26, no. 1 (2000): 51–65.

18 Nagoski, *Come Together*, 29–36.

19 William H. Masters and Virginia E. Johnson, *Human Sexual Response* (Boston: Little, Brown and Company, 1966).

20 Nagoski, *Come Together*, 29–36.

21 John Bancroft and Erick Janssen, "The Dual Control Model of Male Sexual Response: A Theoretical Approach to Centrally Mediated Erectile Dysfunction," *Neuroscience & Biobehavioral Reviews* 24, no. 5 (2000): 571–9.

22 Nagoski, *Come as You Are*, 46–51.

23 Jeff Guenther (@therapyjeff), "For My Men Out There," YouTube Short, August 24, 2022, https://www.youtube.com/shorts/YqjnQvWi96c.

Chapter 7

1 Kathrin F. Stanger-Hall and David W. Hall, "Abstinence-only Education and Teen Pregnancy Rates: Why We Need Comprehensive Sex Education in the US," *PloS one* 6, no. 10 (2011): e24658.

2 Leslie M. Kantor and Laura Lindberg, "Pleasure and Sex Education: The Need for Broadening Both Content and Measurement," *American Journal of Public Health* 110, no. 2 (2020): 145–8.

3 Gilda Sedgh et al., "Adolescent Pregnancy, Birth, and Abortion Rates Across Countries: Levels and Recent Trends," *Journal of Adolescent Health* 56, no. 2 (2015): 223–30; Chelsea L. Shannon and Jeffrey D. Klausner, "The Growing Epidemic of Sexually Transmitted Infections in Adolescents: A Neglected Population," *Current Opinion in Pediatrics* 30, no. 1 (2018): 137–43.

4 Pamela J. Sawyer et al., "Discrimination and the Stress Response: Psychological and Physiological Consequences of Anticipating Prejudice in Interethnic Interactions," *American Journal of Public Health* 102, no. 5 (2012): 1020–6.

5 Monnica Williams, Muna Osman, and Chrysalis Hyon, "Understanding the Psychological Impact of Oppression Using the Trauma Symptoms of Discrimination Scale," *Chronic Stress* 7 (2023): 24705470221149511.

6 MV Lee Badgett, "The Wage Effects of Sexual Orientation Discrimination," *ILR Review* 48, no. 4 (1995): 726–39; Carol Rose DeLilly and Jacquelyn H. Flaskerud, "Discrimination and Health Outcomes," *Issues in Mental Health Nursing* 33, no. 11 (2012): 801–4; David W. Johnston and Grace Lordan, "Discrimination Makes Me Sick! An Examination of the Discrimination–Health Relationship," *Journal of Health Economics* 31, no. 1 (2012): 99–111.

7 Joel R. Anderson et al., "Revisiting the Jezebel Stereotype: The Impact of Target Race on Sexual Objectification," *Psychology of Women Quarterly* 42, no. 4 (2018): 461–76; Katherine Elaine Bliss, "The Sexual Revolution in Mexican Studies: New Perspectives on Gender, Sexuality, and Culture in Modern Mexico," *Latin American Research*

Review 36, no. 1 (2001): 247–85; Lydia X. Z. Brown, "Ableist Shame and Disruptive Bodies: Survivorship at the Intersection of Queer, Trans, and Disabled Existence," in *Religion, Disability, and Interpersonal Violence*, ed. Andy J. Johnson, J. Ruth Nelson, and Emily M. Lund (Switzerland: Springer International Publishing, 2017), 163–78; Jardin N. Dogan et al., "'My Partner Will Think I'm Weak or Overthinking My Pain': How Being Superwoman Inhibits Black Women's Sexual Pain Disclosure to Their Partners," *Culture, Health & Sexuality* 25, no. 5 (2023): 567–81; Jack Harrison, Jaime Grant, and Jody L. Herman, "A Gender not Listed Here: Genderqueers, Gender Rebels, and Otherwise in the National Transgender Discrimination Survey," *LGBTQ Public Policy Journal at the Harvard Kennedy School* 2, no. 1 (2012): 13; Alexandria L. Parsons, Arleigh J. Reichl, and Cory L. Pedersen, "Gendered Ableism: Media Representations and Gender Role Beliefs' Effect on Perceptions of Disability and Sexuality," *Sexuality and Disability* 35 (2017): 207–25; Preeti S. Rawat, "Patriarchal Beliefs, Women's Empowerment, and General Well-being," *Vikalpa* 39, no. 2 (2014): 43–56; Megan Sutter and Paul B. Perrin, "Discrimination, Mental Health, and Suicidal Ideation Among LGBTQ People of Color," *Journal of Counseling Psychology* 63, no. 1 (2016): 98; Clara L. Wilkins et al., "Racial Stereotypes and Interracial Attraction: Phenotypic Prototypicality and Perceived Attractiveness of Asians," *Cultural Diversity and Ethnic Minority Psychology* 17, no. 4 (2011): 427; Rachel Yehuda, A. M. Y. Lehrner, and Talli Y. Rosenbaum, "PTSD and Sexual Dysfunction in Men and Women," *The Journal of Sexual Medicine* 12, no. 5 (2015): 1107–19.

8   Siobhan E. Sutherland, Uzma S. Rehman, and Jackson A. Goodnight, "A Typology of Women with Low Sexual Desire," *Archives of Sexual Behavior* 49, no. 2 (2020): 1–13.

9   Bethany Butzer and Lorne Campbell, "Adult Attachment, Sexual Satisfaction, and Relationship Satisfaction: A Study of Married Couples," *Personal Relationships* 15, no. 1 (2008): 141–54.

10 Ana A. Carvalheira and Pedro Alexandre Costa, "The Impact of Relational Factors on Sexual Satisfaction among Heterosexual and Homosexual Men," *Sexual and Relationship Therapy* 30, no. 3 (2015): 314–24; Kristen P. Mark, Justin R. Garcia, and Helen E. Fisher, "Perceived Emotional and Sexual Satisfaction Across Sexual Relationship Contexts: Gender and Sexual Orientation Differences and Similarities," *The Canadian Journal of Human Sexuality* 24, no. 2 (2015): 120–30; Patrícia Monteiro Pascoal, Isabel Narciso, and Nuno Monteiro Pereira, "Emotional Intimacy is the Best Predictor of Sexual Satisfaction of Men and Women with Sexual Arousal Problems," *International Journal of Impotence Research* 25, no. 2 (2013): 51–5; Dustin K. Shepler et al., "Predictors of Sexual Satisfaction for Partnered Lesbian, Gay, And Bisexual Adults," *Psychology of Sexual Orientation and Gender Diversity* 5, no. 1 (2018): 25; Jessica R. Wood, Robin R. Milhausen, and Nicole K. Jeffrey, "Why Have Sex? Reasons for Having Sex Among Lesbian, Bisexual, Queer, and Questioning Women in Romantic Relationships," *The Canadian Journal of Human Sexuality* 23, no. 2 (2014): 75–88.

11 Esther Perel, *Mating in Captivity: Unlocking Erotic Intelligence* (New York: HarperCollins, 2006).

12 Rhonda N. Balzarini et al., "Eroticism Versus Nurturance: How Eroticism and Nurturance Differs in Polyamorous and Monogamous Relationships," *Social Psychology* 50, no. 3 (2019): 185; Amy C. Moors, Jes L. Matsick, and Heath A. Schechinger, "Unique and Shared Relationship Benefits of Consensually Non-Monogamous and Monogamous Relationships," *European Psychologist* 22, no. 1 (2017): 55–71.

13 Napoleon Hill, *Think and Grow Rich* (Meriden, CT: The Ralston Society, 1937), 260–90.

14 Mark Manson, *The Subtle Art of Not Giving a F*ck: A Counterintuitive Approach to Living a Good Life* (New York: HarperCollins, 2016).

15 Jacquelyn Tenaglia (@no.bs.therapist), "What did I miss?" Instagram post, April 16, 2024, https://www.instagram.com/p/C5OoKBHOEmn/.

Part 3

1 Kathryn E. Flynn et al., "Sexual Satisfaction and the Importance of Sexual Health to Quality of Life Throughout the Life Course of US Adults," *The Journal of Sexual Medicine* 13, no. 11 (2016): 1642–50; Riki E. Slayday et al., "Erectile Function, Sexual Satisfaction, and Cognitive Decline in Men from Midlife to Older Adulthood," *The Gerontologist* 63, no. 2 (2023): 382–94.

2 Sari M. Van Anders et al., "The Heteronormativity Theory of Low Sexual Desire in Women Partnered with Men," *Archives of Sexual Behavior* 51, no. 1 (2022): 391–415.

3 Gary D. Chapman, *The 5 Love Languages: The Secret to Love that Lasts* (Chicago: Northfield, 2010).

Chapter 9

1 Heather A. Rupp and Kim Wallen, "Sex Differences in Response to Visual Sexual Stimuli: A Review," *Archives of Sexual Behavior* 37 (2008): 206–18.

2 Emily Nagoski, "The Truth About Unwanted Arousal," filmed April 2018 at TED2018, Vancouver, British Columbia, video, 15:06, https://www.ted.com/talks/emily_nagoski_the_truth_about_unwanted_arousal.

Chapter 10

1 David A. Frederick et al., "What Keeps Passion Alive? Sexual Satisfaction Is Associated with Sexual Communication, Mood Setting, Sexual Variety, Oral Sex, Orgasm, and Sex Frequency in a National US Study," *The Journal of Sex Research* 54, no. 2 (2017): 186–201.

Chapter 11

1. David A. Frederick et al., "What Keeps Passion Alive? Sexual Satisfaction Is Associated with Sexual Communication, Mood Setting, Sexual Variety, Oral Sex, Orgasm, and Sex Frequency in a National US Study," *The Journal of Sex Research* 54, no. 2 (2017): 186–201.

Chapter 12

1. Sandra Šević, Iva Ivanković, and Aleksandar Štulhofer, "Emotional Intimacy among Coupled Heterosexual and Gay/Bisexual Croatian Men: Assessing the Role of Minority Stress," *Archives of Sexual Behavior* 45 (2016): 1259–68; Jessica R. Wood et al., "Motivations for Engaging in Consensually Non-Monogamous Relationships," *Archives of Sexual Behavior* 50, no. 4 (2021): 1253–72; Hana Yoo et al., "Couple Communication, Emotional and Sexual Intimacy, and Relationship Satisfaction," *Journal of Sex & Marital Therapy* 40, no. 4 (2014): 275–93.

Chapter 13

1. Audre Lorde, "Uses of the Erotic: The Erotic as Power," in *Sister Outsider: Essays and Speeches* (Berkeley, CA: Crossing Press, 2012), 53–9.

2. Charlotta Carlström, "BDSM, Becoming and the Flows of Desire," *Culture, Health & Sexuality* 21, no. 4 (2019): 404–15; Richard A. Sprott, "Reimagining 'Kink': Transformation, Growth, and Healing Through BDSM," *Journal of Humanistic Psychology* (2020): 0022167819900036.

3. Andreas A.J. Wismeijer and Marcel A.L.M. van Assen, "Psychological Characteristics of BDSM Practitioners," *The Journal of Sexual Medicine* 10, no. 8 (2013): 1943–52.

4. Ela Przybylo, *Asexual Erotics: Intimate Readings of Compulsory Sexuality* (Columbus, OH: The Ohio State University Press, 2019).

BIBLIOGRAPHY

Albert, Hanne. "Psychosomatic Group Treatment Helps Women with Chronic Pelvic Pain." *Journal of Psychosomatic Obstetrics & Gynecology* 20, no. 4 (1999): 216–25. https://doi.org/10.3109/01674829909075598.

Alexander, Frederick Matthias. *Man's Supreme Inheritance: Conscious Guidance and Control in Relation to Human Evolution in Civilization*. London: Methuen, 1918.

American Psychiatric Association. *Diagnostic and Statistical Manual of Mental Disorders, Text Revision (5th ed.), DSM-V-TR*. Washington, DC: author, 2000.

American Psychiatric Association. "Sexual Arousal." APA Psychology Dictionary. Last modified April 19, 2018. https://dictionary.apa.org/sexual-arousal.

Anderson, Joel R., Elise Holland, Courtney Heldreth, and Scott P. Johnson. "Revisiting the Jezebel Stereotype: The Impact of Target Race on Sexual Objectification." *Psychology of Women Quarterly* 42, no. 4 (2018): 461–76. https://doi.org/10.1177/0361684318791543.

Apostolou, Menelaos. "Size Did Not Matter: An Evolutionary Account of the Variation in Penis Size and Size Anxiety." *Cogent Psychology* 3, no. 1 (2016): 1147933. https://doi.org/10.1080/23311908.2016.1147933.

Arlinghaus, Katherine R., and Craig A. Johnston, "The Importance of Creating Habits and Routine." *American Journal of Lifestyle Medicine* 13, no. 2 (2019): 142–4. https://doi.org/10.1177/1559827618818044.

Badgett, M.V. Lee. "The Wage Effects of Sexual Orientation Discrimination." *ILR Review* 48, no. 4 (1995): 726–39. https://doi.org/10.2307/2524353.

Balzarini, Rhonda N., Christoffer Dharma, Amy Muise, and Taylor Kohut. "Eroticism Versus Nurturance: How Eroticism and Nurturance Differs in Polyamorous and Monogamous Relationships." *Social Psychology* 50, no. 3 (2019): 185. https://doi.org/10.1027/1864-9335/a000378.

Bancroft, John, and Erick Janssen. "The Dual Control Model of Male Sexual Response: A Theoretical Approach to Centrally Mediated Erectile Dysfunction." *Neuroscience & Biobehavioral Reviews* 24, no. 5 (2000): 571–9. https://doi.org/10.1016/S0149-7634(00)00024-5.

Basran, Giuseppe Fallara, Edoardo Pozzi, Francesco Montorsi, Andrea Salonia et al. "Worldwide Temporal Trends in Penile Length: A Systematic Review and Meta-Analysis." *The World Journal of Men's Health* 41, no. 4 (2023): 848–60. https://doi.org/10.5534/wjmh.220203.

Basson, Rosemary. "The Female Sexual Response: A Different Model." *Journal of Sex &Marital Therapy* 26, no. 1 (2000): 51–65. https://doi.org/10.1080/009262300278641.

Belladelli, Federico, Francesco Del Giudice, Frank Glover, Evan Mulloy, Wade Muncey, Satvir Bliss, and Katherine Elaine. "The Sexual Revolution in Mexican Studies: New

Perspectives on Gender, Sexuality, and Culture in Modern Mexico." *Latin American Research Review* 36, no. 1 (2001): 247–85. https://doi.org/10.1017/S0023879100018926.

Bostan, Cristina Maria. "The Role of Motivational Persistence and Resilience Over the Well-being Changes Registered in Time." *Symposion* 2, no. 2 (2015): 215–41. https://doi.org/10.5840/symposion20152212.

Brotto, Lori A., Rosemary Basson, and Mijal Luria, "A Mindfulness-Based Group Psychoeducational Intervention Targeting Sexual Arousal Disorder in Women." *The Journal of Sexual Medicine* 5, no. 7 (2008): 1646–59. https://doi.org/10.1111/j.1743-6109.2008.00850.x.

Brotto, Lori A., and Emily Nagoski. *Better Sex Through Mindfulness: How Women Can Cultivate Desire*. Vancouver, BC: Greystone Books, 2018.

Brown, Lydia X.Z. "Ableist Shame and Disruptive Bodies: Survivorship at the Intersection of Queer, Trans, and Disabled Existence." In *Religion, Disability, and Interpersonal Violence*, edited by Andy J. Johnson, J. Ruth Nelson, Emily M. Lund, 163–78. Switzerland: Springer International Publishing, 2017. https://doi.org/10.1007/978-3-319-56901-7.

Bryant-Davis, Thema, editor, *Surviving Sexual Violence: A Guide to Recovery and Empowerment*. Lanham, MD: Rowman & Littlefield Publishers, 2011.

Butzer, Bethany, and Lorne Campbell. "Adult Attachment, Sexual Satisfaction, and Relationship Satisfaction: A Study of Married Couples." *Personal Relationships* 15, no. 1 (2008): 141–54. https://doi.org/10.1111/j.1475-6811.2007.00189.x.

Carlström, Charlotta. "BDSM, Becoming and the Flows of Desire." *Culture, Health & Sexuality* 21, no. 4 (2019): 404–15. https://doi.org/10.1080/13691058.2018.1485969.

Carvalheira, Ana A., and Pedro Alexandre Costa. "The Impact of Relational Factors on Sexual Satisfaction Among Heterosexual and Homosexual Men." *Sexual and Relationship Therapy* 30, no. 3 (2015): 314–24. https://doi.org/10.1080/14681994.2015.1041372.

Centers for Disease Control and Prevention (CDC). "How Much Sleep Do I Need?" Sleep and Sleep Disorders. Last modified September 14, 2022. https://www.cdc.gov/sleep/about_sleep/how_much_sleep.html.

Chapman, Gary D. *The Five Love Languages: The Secret to Love That Lasts*. Chicago: Northfield, 2010.

Chivers, Meredith L., Michael C. Seto, Martin L. Lalumière, Ellen Laan, and Teresa Grimbos. "Agreement of Self-Reported and Genital Measures of Sexual Arousal in Men and Women: A Meta-Analysis." *Archives of Sexual Behavior* 39, no. 1 (2010): 5–56. https://doi.org/10.1007/s10508-009-9556-9.

Cobb, Sidney. "Social Support as a Moderator of Life Stress." *Psychosomatic medicine* 38, no. 5 (1976): 300–14. https://doi.org/10.1097/00006842-197609000-00003.

Colle, Kathleen F. Flugel, Ann Vincent, Stephen S. Cha, Laura L. Loehrer, Brent A. Bauer, and Dietlind L. Wahner-Roedler. "Measurement of Quality of Life and Participant Experience with the Mindfulness-based Stress Reduction Program." *Complementary Therapies in Clinical Practice* 16, no. 1 (2010): 30–40. https://doi.org/10.1016/j.ctcp.2009.06.008.

Das, Aniruddha. "Masturbation in the United States." *Journal of Sex & Marital Therapy* 33, no. 4 (2007): 301–17. https://doi.org/10.1080/00926230701385514.

DeLilly, Carol Rose, and Jacquelyn H. Flaskerud. "Discrimination and Health Outcomes." *Issues in Mental Health Nursing* 33, no. 11 (2012): 801–4. https://doi.org/10.3109/01612840.2012.671442.

Demarin, Vida, and Sandra Morović. "Neuroplasticity." *Periodicum Biologorum* 116, no. 2 (2014): 209–11. https://hrcak.srce.hr/126369.

Dinesh, Tantri Keerthi, Ankitha Shetty, Vijay Shree Dhyani, Shwetha TS, and Komal Jenifer Dsouza. "Effectiveness of Mindfulness-based Interventions on Well-being and Work-related Stress in the Financial Sector: A Systematic Review and Meta-Analysis Protocol." *Systematic Reviews* 11, no. 1 (2022): 79. https://doi.org/10.1186/s13643-022-01956-x.

Dogan, Jardin N., Shemeka Y. Thorpe, Natalie Malone, Jasmine Jester, Danelle Stevens-Watkins, and Candice Hargons. "'My Partner Will Think I'm Weak or Overthinking My Pain': How Being Superwoman Inhibits Black Women's Sexual Pain Disclosure to Their Partners." *Culture, Health & Sexuality* 25, no. 5 (2023): 567–81. https://doi.org/10.1080/13691058.2022.2072956.

Dussault, Éliane, Mylène Fernet, and Natacha Godbout. "A Metasynthesis of Qualitative Studies on Mindfulness, Sexuality, and Relationality." *Mindfulness* 11, no. 12 (2020): 2682–94. https://doi.org/10.1007/s12671-020-01463-x.

Dweck, Carol S. *Mindset: The New Psychology of Success*. New York: Random House, 2006.

Fava, Giovanni A., Fiammetta Cosci, and Nicoletta Sonino. "Current Psychosomatic Practice." *Psychotherapy and Psychosomatics* 86, no. 1 (2017): 13–30. https://doi.org/10.1159/000448856.

Flynn, Kathryn E., Li Lin, Deborah Watkins Bruner, Jill M. Cyranowski, Elizabeth A. Hahn, Diana D. Jeffery, Jennifer Barsky Reese, Bryce B. Reeve, Rebecca A. Shelby, and Kevin P. Weinfurt. "Sexual Satisfaction and the Importance of Sexual Health to Quality of Life Throughout the Life Course of US Adults." *The Journal of Sexual Medicine* 13, no. 11 (2016): 1642–50. https://doi.org/10.1016/j.jsxm.2016.08.011.

Frederick, David A., Janet Lever, Brian Joseph Gillespie, and Justin R. Garcia. "What Keeps Passion Alive? Sexual Satisfaction is Associated with Sexual Communication, Mood Setting, Sexual Variety, Oral Sex, Orgasm, and Sex Frequency in a National US Study." *The Journal of Sex Research* 54, no. 2 (2017): 186–201. https://doi.org/10.1080/00224499.2015.1137854.

Gollwitzer, Peter M. "Implementation Intentions: Strong Effects of Simple Plans." *American Psychologist* 54, no. 7 (1999): 493–503. https://doi.org/10.1037/0003-066X.54.7.493.

Gozalo-Pascual, Rodrigo, Héctor González-Ordi, María Ángeles Atín-Arratibel, Javier Llames-Sánchez, and Ángela C. Álvarez-Melcón. "Efficacy of the Myofascial Approach as a Manual Therapy Technique in Patients with Clinical Anxiety: A Randomized Controlled Clinical Trial." *Complementary Therapies in Clinical Practice* 51 (2023): 101753. https://doi.org/10.1016/j.ctcp.2023.101753.

Guenther, Jeff (@therapyjeff). "For My Men Out There." YouTube Short, August 24, 2022, https://www.youtube.com/shorts/YqjnQvWi96c.

Hanna, Thomas, "The Field of Somatics." *Somatics* 1, no. 1 (1976): 30–4.
Harrison, Jack, Jaime Grant, and Jody L. Herman. "A Gender not Listed Here: Genderqueers, Gender Rebels, and Otherwise in the National Transgender Discrimination Survey." *LGBTQ Public Policy Journal at the Harvard Kennedy School* 2, no. 1 (2012): 13.
Herbenick, Debby, Tsung-Chieh Fu, Jennifer Arter, Stephanie A. Sanders, and Brian Dodge. "Women's Experiences with Genital Touching, Sexual Pleasure, and Orgasm: Results from a US Probability Sample of Women Ages 18 to 94." *Journal of Sex & Marital Therapy* 44, no. 2 (2018): 201–12. https://doi.org/10.1080/0092623X.2017.1346530
Hill, Napoleon. *Think and Grow Rich*. Meriden, CT: The Ralston Society, 1937.
Johnston, David W., and Grace Lordan. "Discrimination Makes Me Sick! An Examination of the Discrimination–health Relationship." *Journal of Health Economics* 31, no. 1 (2012): 99–111. https://doi.org/10.1016/j.jhealeco.2011.12.002.
Kames, Linda D., Andrea J. Rapkin, Bruce D. Naliboff, Simin Afifi, and Theresa Ferrer-Brechner. "Effectiveness of an Interdisciplinary Pain Management Program for the Treatment of Chronic Pelvic Pain." *Pain* 41, no. 1 (1990): 41–6. https://doi.org/10.1016/0304-3959(90)91107-T.
Kantor, Leslie M., and Laura Lindberg. "Pleasure and Sex Education: The Need for Broadening Both Content and Measurement." *American Journal of Public Health* 110, no. 2 (2020): 145–8. https://doi.org/10.2105/AJPH.2019.305320.
Kessler, Anna, Sam Sollie, Ben Challacombe, Karen Briggs, and Mieke Van Hemelrijck. "The Global Prevalence of Erectile Dysfunction: A Review." *BJU International* 124, no. 4 (2019): 587–99. https://doi.org/10.1111/bju.14813.
Khoury, Bassam, Manoj Sharma, Sarah E. Rush, and Claude Fournier. "Mindfulness-based Stress Reduction for Healthy Individuals: A Meta-Analysis." *Journal of Psychosomatic Research* 78, no. 6 (2015): 519–28. https://doi.org/10.1016/j.jpsychores.2015.03.009.
Kuhfuß, Marie, Tobias Maldei, Andreas Hetmanek, and Nicola Baumann. "Somatic Experiencing: Effectiveness and Key Factors of a Body-Oriented Trauma Therapy: A Scoping Literature Review." *European Journal of Psychotraumatology* 12, no. 1 (2021): 1929023. https://doi.org/10.1080/20008198.2021.1929023.
Lally, Phillippa, Cornelia H.M. Van Jaarsveld, Henry W.W. Potts, and Jane Wardle. "How Are Habits Formed: Modelling Habit Formation in the Real World." *European Journal of Social Psychology* 40, no. 6 (2010): 998–1009. https://doi.org/10.1002/ejsp.674.
Lamvu, Georgine, Jorge Carrillo, Chensi Ouyang, and Andrea Rapkin. "Chronic Pelvic Pain in Women: A Review." *Jama* 325, no. 23 (2021): 2381–91. doi:10.1001/jama.2021.2631.
Leavitt, Chelom E., Eva S. Lefkowitz, and Emily A. Waterman. "The Role of Sexual Mindfulness in Sexual Wellbeing, Relational Wellbeing, and Self-Esteem." *Journal of Sex & Marital Therapy* 45, no. 6 (2019): 497–509. https://doi.org/10.1080/0092623X.2019.1572680.
Lehmiller, Justin J., Justin R. Garcia, Amanda N. Gesselman, and Kristen P. Mark. "Less Sex, but More Sexual Diversity: Changes in Sexual Behavior During the COVID-19

Coronavirus Pandemic." *Leisure Sciences* 43, no. 1–2 (2020): 295–304. https://doi.org/10.1080/01490400.2020.1774016.

Leonard, Ashley. "An Investigation of Masturbation and Coping Style." Presentation at 38th Annual Western Pennsylvania Undergraduate Psychology Conference, Slippery Rock University, 2010.

Levin, Roy J. "Sexual Activity, Health and Well-being–the Beneficial Roles of Coitus and Masturbation." *Sexual and Relationship Therapy* 22, no. 1 (2007): 135–48. https://doi.org/10.1080/14681990601149197.

Levine, Glenn N., Elaine E. Steinke, Faisal G. Bakaeen, Biykem Bozkurt, Melvin D. Cheitlin, Jamie Beth Conti, Elyse Foster, Tiny Jaarsma, Robert A. Kloner, Richard A. Lange, et al. "Sexual Activity and Cardiovascular Disease: A Scientific Statement from the American Heart Association." *Circulation* 125, no. 8 (2012): 1058–72. https://doi.org/10.1161/CIR.0b013e3182447787.

Levine, Peter A. "Accumulated Stress, Reserve Capacity, and Disease." PhD diss., University of California, Berkeley, 1976, 1–24.

Levine, Peter A. *Healing Trauma: The Innate Capacity to Transform Overwhelming Experiences.* Berkely, CA: North Atlantic Books, 1997.

Levine, Peter A. *Waking the Tiger: Healing Trauma: The Innate Capacity to Transform Overwhelming Experiences.* Berkeley, CA: North Atlantic Books, 1997.

Lorde, Audre. "Uses of the Erotic: The Erotic as Power." In *Sister Outsider: Essays and Speeches*, 53–9. Berkeley, CA: Crossing Press, 2012.

MacDonald, Geoff, and Mark R. Leary. "Why Does Social Exclusion Hurt? The Relationship Between Social and Physical Pain." *Psychological Bulletin* 131, no. 2 (2005): 202. https://doi.org/10.1037/0033-2909.131.2.202.

Mahar, Elizabeth A., Laurie B. Mintz, and Brianna M. Akers. "Orgasm Equality: Scientific Findings and Societal Implications." *Current Sexual Health Reports* 12, no. 1 (2020): 24–32. https://doi.org/10.1007/s11930-020-00237-9.

Manson, Mark. *The Subtle Art of Not Giving a F*ck: A Counterintuitive Approach to Living a Good Life.* New York: HarperCollins, 2016.

Mark, Kristen P., Justin R. Garcia, and Helen E. Fisher. "Perceived Emotional and Sexual Satisfaction Across Sexual Relationship Contexts: Gender and sexual orientation differences and similarities." *The Canadian Journal of Human Sexuality* 24, no. 2 (2015): 120–30. https://doi.org/10.3138/cjhs.242-A8.

Marsiglio, William, and Frank L. Mott. "The Impact of Sex Education on Sexual Activity, Contraceptive Use and Premarital Pregnancy Among American Teenagers." *Family Planning Perspectives* 18, no. 4 (1986): 151–62. https://doi.org/10.2307/2135324.

Masters, William H., and Virginia E. Johnson. *Human Sexual Response.* Boston: Little, Brown and Company, 1966.

McCabe, Marita P., Ira D. Sharlip, Ron Lewis, Elham Atalla, Richard Balon, Alessandra D. Fisher, Edward Laumann, Sun Won Lee, and Robert T. Segraves. "Incidence and Prevalence of Sexual Dysfunction in Women and Men: A Consensus Statement from the Fourth International Consultation on Sexual Medicine 2015." *The Journal of Sexual Medicine* 13, no. 2 (2016): 144–52. https://doi.org/10.1016/j.jsxm.2015.12.034.

Menakem, Resmaa. *My Grandmother's Hands: Racialized Trauma and the Pathway to Mending Our Hearts and Bodies*. Las Vegas: Central Recovery Press, 2017.

Merwin, Kathleen E., and Natalie O. Rosen. "Perceived Partner Responsiveness Moderates the Associations Between Sexual Talk and Sexual and Relationship Well-being in Individuals in Long-term Relationships." *The Journal of Sex Research* (2019): 351–64. https://doi.org/10.1080/00224499.2019.1610151.

Miller-Karas, Elaine. *Building Resilience to Trauma: The Trauma and Community Resiliency Models*. 2nd ed. New York: Routledge, 2023.

Moors, Amy C., Jes L. Matsick, and Heath A. Schechinger. "Unique and Shared Relationship Benefits of Consensually Non-monogamous and Monogamous Relationships." *European Psychologist* 22, no. 1 (2017). https://doi.org/10.1027/1016-9040/a000278

Mrazek, Alissa J., Elliott D. Ihm, Daniel C. Molden, Michael D. Mrazek, Claire M. Zedelius, and Jonathan W. Schooler. "Expanding Minds: Growth Mindsets of Self-Regulation and the Influences on Effort and Perseverance." *Journal of Experimental Social Psychology* 79 (2018): 164–80. https://doi.org/10.1016/j.jesp.2018.07.003.

Nagoski, Emily. *Come as You Are: The Surprising New Science that Will Transform Your Sex Life*. New York: Simon & Schuster, 2015.

Nagoski, Emily. *Come Together: The Science (and Art!) of Creating Lasting Sexual Connections*. New York: Ballantine Books, 2024.

Nagoski, Emily. "The Truth About Unwanted Arousal." Filmed April 2018 at TED2018, Vancouver, British Columbia. Video, 15:06. https://www.ted.com/talks/emily_nagoski_the_truth_about_unwanted_arousal.

Netflix. "All Vulvas are Beautiful." Accessed May 11, 2024. https://www.all-vulvas-are-beautiful.com/.

Nummenmaa, Lauri, Juulia T. Suvilehto, Enrico Glerean, Pekka Santtila, and Jari K. Hietanen. "Topography of Human Erogenous Zones." *Archives of Sexual Behavior* 45 (2016): 1207–16. https://doi.org/10.1007/s10508-016-0745-z.

Ogden, Pat, Kekuni Minton, and Clare Pain. *Trauma and the Body: A Sensorimotor Approach to Psychotherapy*. New York: WW Norton & Company, 2006.

Olson, Jeff. *The Slight Edge: Turning Simple Disciplines into Massive Success and Happiness*. Austin, TX: Greenleaf Book Group, 2013.

Ostrzenski, Adam. "G-Spot Anatomy: A New Discovery." *The Journal of Sexual Medicine* 9, no. 5 (2012): 1355–9. https://doi.org/10.1111/j.1743-6109.2012.02668.x.

Parsons, Alexandria L., Arleigh J. Reichl, and Cory L. Pedersen. "Gendered Ableism: Media Representations and Gender Role Beliefs' Effect on Perceptions of Disability and Sexuality." *Sexuality and Disability* 35 (2017): 207–25. https://doi.org/10.1007/s11195-016-9464-6.

Pascoal, Patrícia Monteiro, Isabel Narciso, and Nuno Monteiro Pereira. "Emotional Intimacy is the Best Predictor of Sexual Satisfaction of Men and Women with Sexual Arousal Problems." *International Journal of Impotence Research* 25, no. 2 (2013): 51–5. https://doi.org/10.1038/ijir.2012.38.

Perel, Esther. *Mating in Captivity Unlocking Erotic Intelligence*. New York: HarperCollins, 2006.

Prause, N., H. Cohen, and G. J. Siegle. "Effects of Adverse Childhood Experiences on Partnered Sexual Arousal Appear Context Dependent." *Sexual and Relationship Therapy* 38, no. 3 (2023): 479–94. https://doi.org/10.1080/14681994.2021.1991907.

Prendergast, Stephanie A., and Elizabeth H. Rummer. *Pelvic Pain Explained: What Everyone Needs to Know.* Lanham, MD: Rowman & Littlefield Publishers: 2017.

Przybylo, Ela. *Asexual Erotics: Intimate Readings of Compulsory Sexuality.* Columbus, OH: The Ohio State University Press, 2019.

Puppo, Vincenzo, and Ilan Gruenwald. "Does the G-Spot Exist? A Review of the Current Literature." *International Urogynecology Journal* 23 (2012): 1665–9. https://doi.org/10.1007/s00192-012-1831-y.

Rawat, Preeti S. "Patriarchal Beliefs, Women's Empowerment, and General Well-Being." *Vikalpa* 39, no. 2 (2014): 43–56. https://doi.org/10.1177/0256090920140206.

Ray, Oakley. "How the Mind Hurts and Heals the Body." *American Psychologist* 59, no. 1 (2004): 29–40. https://doi.org/10.1037/0003-066X.59.1.29.

Rechtschaffen, Allan. "Current Perspectives on the Function of Sleep." *Perspectives in Biology and Medicine* 41, no. 3 (1998): 359–90. https://doi.org/10.1353/pbm.1998.0051.

Rolf, Ida P. *Rolfing: Reestablishing the Natural Alignment and Structural Integration of the Human Body for Vitality and Well-being.* New York: Simon & Schuster, 1989.

Rosen, Raymond C. "Prevalence and Risk Factors of Sexual Dysfunction in Men and Women." *Current Psychiatry Reports* 2, no. 3 (June 2000): 189–95. https://doi.org/10.1007/s11920-996-0006-2.

Rupp, Heather A. and Wallen, Kim. "Sex Differences in Response to Visual Sexual Stimuli: A Review." *Archives of Sexual Behavior* 37 (2008): 206–18. https://doi.org/10.1007/s10508-007-9217-9.

Salisu, Isyaku, Norashidah Hashim, Munir Shehu Mashi, and Hamza Galadanchi Aliyu. "Perseverance of Effort and Consistency of Interest for Entrepreneurial Career Success: Does Resilience Matter?" *Journal of Entrepreneurship in Emerging Economies* 12, no. 2 (2020): 279–304. https://doi.org/10.1108/JEEE-02-2019-0025.

Sawyer, Pamela J., Brenda Major, Bettina J. Casad, Sarah S.M. Townsend, and Wendy Berry Mendes. "Discrimination and the Stress Response: Psychological and Physiological Consequences of Anticipating Prejudice in Interethnic Interactions." *American Journal of Public Health* 102, no. 5 (2012): 1020–6. https://doi.org/10.2105/AJPH.2011.300620.

Schwarzer, Ralf, and Reinhard Fuchs. "Self-Efficacy and Health Behaviours." In *Predicting Health Behaviour*, edited by Mark Conner and Paul Norman, 163–96. Buckingham: Open University Press, 1996.

Sedgh, Gilda, Lawrence B. Finer, Akinrinola Bankole, Michelle A. Eilers, and Susheela Singh. "Adolescent Pregnancy, Birth, and Abortion Rates Across Countries: Levels and Recent Trends." *Journal of Adolescent Health* 56, no. 2 (2015): 223–30. https://doi.org/10.1016/j.jadohealth.2014.09.007

Šević, Sandra, Iva Ivanković, and Aleksandar Štulhofer. "Emotional Intimacy Among Coupled Heterosexual and Gay/Bisexual Croatian Men: Assessing the Role of Minority Stress." *Archives of Sexual Behavior* 45 (2016): 1259–68. https://doi.org/10.1007/s10508-015-0538-9.

Shannon, Chelsea L., and Jeffrey D. Klausner. "The Growing Epidemic of Sexually Transmitted Infections in Adolescents: A Neglected Population." *Current Opinion in Pediatrics* 30, no. 1 (2018): 137–43. https://doi.org/10.1097/MOP.0000000000000578.

Shepler, Dustin K., Jared M. Smendik, Kate M. Cusick, and David R. Tucker. "Predictors of Sexual Satisfaction for Partnered Lesbian, Gay, and Bisexual Adults." *Psychology of Sexual Orientation and Gender Diversity* 5, no. 1 (2018): 25. https://doi.org/10.1037/sgd0000252.

Slayday, Riki E., Tyler R. Bell, Michael J. Lyons, Teresa S. Warren, Rosemary Toomey, Richard Vandiver, Martin J. Sliwinski, William S. Kremen, and Carol E. Franz. "Erectile Function, Sexual Satisfaction, and Cognitive Decline in Men from Midlife to Older Adulthood." *The Gerontologist* 63, no. 2 (2023): 382–94. https://doi.org/10.1093/geront/gnac151.

Sprott, Richard A. "Reimagining 'Kink': Transformation, Growth, and Healing Through BDSM." *Journal of Humanistic Psychology* (2020): 0022167819900036. https://doi.org/10.1177/0022167819900036.

Stanger-Hall, Kathrin F., and David W. Hall. "Abstinence-Only Education and Teen Pregnancy Rates: Why We Need Comprehensive Sex Education in the US." *PloS one* 6, no. 10 (2011): e24658. https://doi.org/10.1371/journal.pone.0024658.

Strachan, Ellie, and Betty Staples. "Masturbation." *Pediatrics in Review* 33, no. 4 (2012): 190–1. https://doi.org/10.1542/pir.33-4-190.

Sutherland, Siobhan E., Uzma S. Rehman, and Jackson A. Goodnight. "A Typology of Women with Low Sexual Desire." *Archives of Sexual Behavior* (2020): 1–13. https://doi.org/10.1007/s10508-020-01805-9.

Sutter, Megan, and Paul B. Perrin. "Discrimination, Mental Health, and Suicidal Ideation Among LGBTQ People of Color." *Journal of Counseling Psychology* 63, no. 1 (2016): 98. https://doi.org/10.1037/cou0000126.

Tenaglia, Jacquelyn (@no.bs.therapist). "What did I miss?" Instagram post, April 16, 2024. https://www.instagram.com/p/C50oKBHOEmn/.

Tengland, Per-Anders. "Behavior Change or Empowerment: On the Ethics of Health-promotion Strategies." *Public Health Ethics* 5, no. 2 (2012): 140–53. https://doi.org/10.1093/phe/phs022.

Thorpe, Shemeka, Natalie Malone, Rayven L. Peterson, Praise Iyiewuare, Monyae Kerney, and Candice N. Hargons. "Black Queer Women's Pleasure: A Review." *Current Sexual Health Reports* 15, no. 2 (2023): 100–6. https://doi.org/10.1007/s11930-023-00357-y.

Uloko, Maria, Erika P. Isabey, and Blair R. Peters. "How Many Nerve Fibers Innervate the Human Glans Clitoris: A Histomorphometric Evaluation of the Dorsal Nerve of the Clitoris." *The Journal of Sexual Medicine* 20, no. 3 (2023): 247–52. https://doi.org/10.1093/jsxmed/qdac027.

van Anders, Sari M., Debby Herbenick, Lori A. Brotto, Emily A. Harris, and Sara B. Chadwick. "The Heteronormativity Theory of Low Sexual Desire in Women Partnered with Men." *Archives of Sexual Behavior* 51, no. 1 (2022): 391–415. https://doi.org/10.1007/s10508-021-02100-x.

Van der Kolk, Bessel A. *The Body Keeps the Score: Brain, Mind, and Body in the Healing of Trauma*. New York: Penguin Books, 2014.

Wilkins, Clara L., Joy F. Chan, and Cheryl R. Kaiser. "Racial Stereotypes and Interracial Attraction: Phenotypic Prototypicality and Perceived Attractiveness of Asians." *Cultural Diversity and Ethnic Minority Psychology* 17, no. 4 (2011): 427. https://doi.org/10.1037/a0024733.

Williams, Monnica, Muna Osman, and Chrysalis Hyon. "Understanding the Psychological Impact of Oppression Using the Trauma Symptoms of Discrimination Scale." *Chronic Stress* 7 (2023): 24705470221149511. https://doi.org/10.1177/24705470221149511

Wismeijer, Andreas A.J., and Marcel A.L.M. van Assen. "Psychological Characteristics of BDSM Practitioners." *The Journal of Sexual Medicine* 10, no. 8 (2013): 1943–52. https://doi.org/10.1111/jsm.12192.

Wood, Jessica R., Robin R. Milhausen, and Nicole K. Jeffrey. "Why Have Sex? Reasons for Having Sex Among Lesbian, Bisexual, Queer, and Questioning Women in Romantic Relationships." *The Canadian Journal of Human Sexuality* 23, no. 2 (2014): 75–88. https://doi.org/10.3138/cjhs.2592.

Wood, Jessica R., Carm De Santis, Serge Desmarais, and Robin Milhausen. "Motivations for Engaging in Consensually Non-Monogamous Relationships." *Archives of Sexual Behavior* 50, no. 4 (2021): 1253–72. https://doi.org/10.1007/s10508-020-01873-x.

World Health Organization. "What is Stress?" Stress, 2023, Last modified February 21, 2023. https://www.who.int/news-room/questions-and-answers/item/stress.

Worrall, Hugh, Richard Schweizer, Ellen Marks, Lin Yuan, Chris Lloyd, and Rob Ramjan. "The Effectiveness of Support Groups: A Literature Review." *Mental Health and Social Inclusion* 22, no. 2 (2018): 85–93. https://doi.org/10.1108/MHSI-12-2017-0055.

Wu, Tingting, Alexander J. Dufford, Melissa-Ann Mackie, Laura J. Egan, and Jin Fan. "The Capacity of Cognitive Control Estimated from a Perceptual Decision Making Task." *Scientific Reports* 6, no. 1 (2016): 34025. https://doi.org/10.1038/srep34025.

Yehuda, Rachel, A. M. Y. Lehrner, and Talli Y. Rosenbaum. "PTSD and Sexual Dysfunction in Men and Women." *The Journal of Sexual Medicine* 12, no. 5 (2015): 1107–19. https://doi.org/10.1111/jsm.12856.

Yoo, Hana, Suzanne Bartle-Haring, Randal D. Day, and Rashmi Gangamma. "Couple Communication, Emotional and Sexual Intimacy, and Relationship Satisfaction." *Journal of Sex & Marital Therapy* 40, no. 4 (2014): 275–93. https://doi.org/10.1080/0092623X.2012.751072.

Zhang, Jianzhong, ChaoZhao Liang, Xuejun Shang, and Hongjun Li. "Chronic Prostatitis/Chronic Pelvic Pain Syndrome: A Disease or Symptom? Current Perspectives on Diagnosis, Treatment, And Prognosis." *American Journal of Men's Health* 14, no. 1 (2020): 1557988320903200. https://doi.org/10.1177/1557988320903200.

INDEX

Note: Page numbers in *italics* refer to figures; page numbers followed by 'n' indicate note numbers.

AAPI Women Lead 273
acroyoga 22, 23, 156, 236
active listening 256
ADDitude Magazine 271
Afrosexology 273
"All Vulvas Are Beautiful" 110, 281 n.5
alternative possibilities 33, 88, 96–9, 166, 168
AMAB, *see* assigned male at birth (AMAB)
Amy 158–9
anal stimulation 122
anus 58, 111, 122–3
anxiety 1, 2, 9, 24, 27, 28, 30, 33, 35, 42, 44, 45, 47, 58, 69, 75, 78, 82, 87, 91, 93, 103, 107, 111, 112, 115, 127, 130, 138–9, 151, 154, 155, 173, 175, 206, 215, 219, 235, 270
  performance 2, 42, 58, 75, 151, 214
  sexual 27, 78, 87, 91
API Queer Women and Transgender Community (APIQWTC) 273
APIQWTC, *see* API Queer Women and Transgender Community (APIQWTC)
aromantics 272
arousal 2–7, 9, 16–18, 22, 75, 76, 101, 143, 153, 177–8, 182, 185–7, 191, 202, 209, 225, 227, 235, 240, 249, 270
Arousal Architecture® 3, 5, 71, 76, 95, 122, 125, 130, 132, 133, 135, 153, 159, 166, 173–5
  applications of 185–7, 243, 249–50

assessment 177, 179–80, 182, 185, 188, *189*, 194–9, 207, 249
design and exploration 243–8, *245–7*
dimensions of 179–82, 185, 188, *189*, 190, 192, 194, 201, 203–5, 209, 233, 235, 243, 253
dynamic model 188–90, *189*
Embodied Experience dimension 180, 183, 190, 193, 195–6, 205, 209–15, 217, 221, 228, 244, 251
Energetic Connection dimension 180, 183, 190, 193, 197–8, 205, 223–9, 234, 244
Erotic Exploration dimension 180, 183, 190, 198–9, 211, 231–42, 244
examples 182–5, *183*, *184*, 202, 210, 219, 225, 233, 237–8, 244, *245*, *246*
implementation of 249–50
Mental Headspace dimension 180, 181, 183, 186, 190, 196–7, 205, 217–22, 228, 244, 251, 256
phrases of 178–9
responsive desire 191–2, 203, 211, 264
results 177, 179–85, *183*, *184*, 188, 189, 194, 204, 205, 207, 213, 218, 244, 249, 251
Sexual Aversion Cycle 183, 184, 190–1
sexual pleasure 6, 178, 187, 192–3
Sexual Stimulation dimension 180, 183, 190, 194–5, 201–8, 211, 244
small wins 193–4

INDEX

threat response 174, 190–1
arousal language 6, 178–80, 185, 187, 191, 192, 202–4, 211–12, 219–20, 225–7, 239–40, 243
arousal non-concordance 126, 127, 208
Asexual Agenda 272
asexuality 272
assigned male at birth (AMAB) 114, 116, 208
Attention Deficit Hyperactivity Disorder 147, 186
authentic arousal (and pleasure) 3, 5, 10, 55, 174, 179, 225, 231, 252
authentic sexual wellness 17
automatic thought 72–3, 98, 99, 167, 168, 172

Bancroft, J. 283 n.21
"Dual Control Model of Sexual Response" 130
BDSM (bondage and discipline, dominance and submission, sadism and masochism) 153, 154, 210, 219, 224, 231, 233, 234, 241, 286 n.2, 286 n.3
Beducated 272
beliefs 24, 41, 44, 55–6, 91, 103, 106, 115, 119, 122, 132, 144, 146, 154, 159, 166–8, 171, 232, 265, 266, 284–5 n.7
    cognitive 17
    Empowered Beliefs 57, 70, 73–4
    Limiting Beliefs 70, 73, 74, 98, 221
    mindset 59–66
    negative 11, 18
    outdated 16–19, 63, 69, 94, 96, 98, 99
    political 193
belief systems 3–4, 17–19, 24, 52, 60, 62, 64, 93, 97, 102, 115, 121, 123, 134, 141, 145, 147, 157, 158, 164, 178, 193, 220, 232, 234
    discriminatory 149
    harmful 44, 72, 110, 112, 114, 182
    oppressive 25, 57, 114

outdated 20, 28, 44, 59, 61, 71, 80, 81, 85, 96, 114, 130, 132
and sexual resilience 55–9, 65, 66
Bella 238
Ben 182–5
Bethany 60–2
"Big T" Traumas 89–92
biological sex 4, 108, 109, 113, 116, 119
birth control 12
Black Female Therapists Directory 273
Black Girls' Guide to Surviving Menopause 274
"Black Lives Matter Meditations" 274
Black Women's Pleasure Mapping 274
Body Scanwich 48–50
brain 4, 7, 11, 15, 18, 19, 25–6, 34, 41–3, 49–51, 60, 62–3, 67, 71, 75–6, 107, 117, 123, 124, 126, 144, 157, 166, 178, 211, 217, 220, 236, 271
    neuropathways 4, 5, 84
    neuroplasticity 19, 279 n.1 (chapter 1)
    pathways 5, 8, 21, 24, 28, 32, 33, 35, 55, 61, 67, 69, 70, 72, 77–99, 105, 152, 161, 168, 169, 171, 172, 193, 205
Brathwaite, B.
    Kimbritive 274

Calm app 271
CBT, *see* cognitive behavioral therapy (CBT)
chest 27, 28, 31, 47, 98, 121–2
circumcision 112
cisgender 4, 101, 108, 116, 120, 153
clitoral hood 110, 112
clitoris *109*, 110, 117–20, *118*, *119*, 282 n.8
CNM, *see* consensually non-monogamous (CNM)
cognitive behavioral therapy (CBT) 23, 166–7
cognitive and somatic reframe 165–9, *167*, *169*, 170, 172, 221, 240
cognitive restructuring 166–7

communication   104, 124, 146, 149, 155, 218, 219, 278 n.2, 285 n.1 (chapter 10), 286 n.1 (chapter 11)
   formula   6, 265–6
   issues   150
   levels of   263–4
   skills   88
   strategies   222, 249, 261
   toolbox, building   261–5
   tools   153, 154, 206, 221, 261
compassion   36, 47, 50, 56, 63, 64, 77, 88, 96, 97, 105, 116, 132, 135, 136, 138, 139, 155, 168, 177, 193, 215, 224, 257, 262
   compassionate script   72–3, 221
   non-judgmental   81
   self-compassion   44
Compliment Sandwich   264–5
consensually non-monogamous (CNM)   153–4, 224, 226, 227, 285 n.12
COVID-19 pandemic   2, 278 n.3
Cox, L.   101
couple's pleasure program   183
Cross, L.   274
curiosity   34, 63–4, 69, 95, 104, 177, 246

Dale, B.   274
dating   6, 84, 86, 152, 154–5, 169, 184, 192, 252, 254, 261
   scripts   266–7
depression   2, 45, 124, 155, 220, 235, 240, 275
dirty talk   220, 221, 255–7, 264
discomfort   11, 34–5, 51, 66, 71, 96, 102, 103, 124, 138, 144, 162, 184, 201, 210, 258
   emotional   33
discrimination   115, 146–9, 283 n.4, 283 n.5, 283 n.6, 284 n.7
disgust   102, 105
dissociate   9, 50
distress   35, 62, 90, 138, 149, 153
   clinical   12, 155
   tolerance   36
Dogan-Dixon, J.   274
Dweck, C.   55, 280 n.1 (chapter 4)
dyspareunia   182
dysregulate(d)   9, 87, 88, 95, 98, 99

effective communication   88, 124, 146, 206, 218, 219, 222
Embodied Experience dimension, *see* Arousal Architecture®: Embodied Experience dimension
embodied self-awareness   79–81
EMDR, *see* Eye Movement Desensitization and Reprocessing (EMDR)
emotional resilience   29
Empowered Beliefs   70
   identification of   73–4
empowerment   35, 36, 69, 76, 81, 91, 103, 121, 159, 169, 203, 236, 237, 259, 269, 280 n.6, 284 n.7
Energetic Connection dimension, *see* Arousal Architecture®: Energetic Connection dimension
erectile variability   26, 75, 137, 278 n.1 (chapter 1), 283 n.21, 285 n.1 (part 3)
erection   16, 60, 62, 67, 68, 88, 89, 106, 114, 126, 128, 142, 206
erotic, definition of   232
Erotic Exploration dimension, *see* Arousal Architecture®: Erotic Exploration dimension
Erotic Management   235
Expanded Non-Linear Sexual Response Cycle   130–2, *131*
external genitalia   108–17, *111*, *119*
Eye Movement Desensitization and Reprocessing (EMDR)   24

factual knowledge   16
faith-based counseling and education   274
fixed mindset   56, 68
flirting   133, 134, 150, 152, 153, 165, 224, 228, 255–7

INDEX

foreplay 133, 136
foreskin *111*, 112

gender 109, 127, 134, 136, 147, 149, 233, 274, 283 n.7, 284 n.10
   cisgender 4, 101, 108, 116, 120, 153
   diverse folks, pleasure for 115–17
   identity 113, 117
   sex *vs.* 112–15
   roles 114, 179, 232
   transgender 273, 284 n.7
genital stimulation 78, 137, 165, 202
GoLove CBD Intimate Serum 271
growth mindset 4, 12, 13, 16, 55–7, 67, 68, 70–2, 159
growth-oriented environments 67–8
G-spot 121, 124, 282 n.11
Guenther, J. 133, 283 n.23
guilt-shame spiral 20, 64, 157–8, 169

Hargon, C. N. 274
Hart, E.
   Hoodrat to Headwrap 274
Headspace app 271
healthcare provider(s) 2, 6, 77, 214, 250
   sexual challenges with 258–9
Helfer, N. 274
Hill, N.
   Think and Grow Rich 155, 285 n.13
holistic approach 5, 76
holistic identity 179
holistic sexual wellness 141–72
homologous structures 120
honeymoon phase 19, 60, 151
hormone-mediated vulvodynia 12
Huggins, K.
   Kimbritive 274

iChill app 271
Indigenous peoples resources 275
inner labia (labia minora) 109, 110
International Pelvic Pain Society 271
It Gets Better 273

Jackie 151–3
James 238
Janssen, E.
   "Dual Control Model of Sexual Response" 130, 283 n.21
Jason 126–7
Jessi 182–5, 188
Jessica 107–8
John 60–2

Kate 190
kindness 63–4
kinky 122, 123, 153–4, 232–4, 238, 239, 241, 253, 254, *254*

Latino Network 274
learned responses 17–20, 24, 35, 62, 85, 86, 93, 144
Levine, Peter A. 279 n.1 (chapter 2)
   Waking the Tiger 23, 279 n.2
Limiting Beliefs, identification of 70, 73, 74, 98, 221
linear model of sexual arousal 128, *128*, 129
"little t" traumas 89–91
Lorals 272
Lorde, A.
   "Uses of the Erotic: The Erotic as Power" 232–3, 286 n.1 (chapter 13)
Love Languages® 6, 175, 178, 187
love letter 197, 228, 254–5
low libido 12, 67, 75
low self-esteem 226
lubrication 16, 88, 106, 126, 128, 206

McCabe, J. 271
Malone, N.
   Hoodrat to Headwrap 274
Manson, M.
   *Subtle Art of Not Giving a F*ck, The* 156, 285 n.14
masturbation 66, 102, 103, 157, 201, 281 n.1 (chapter 6), 281 n.2 (chapter 6)

meditation   21, 41, 42, 47, 52, 210, 214
Melt: Massage for Couples   272
Menakem, R.
   My Grandmother's Hands   23, 279 n.2
Mental Headspace dimension, *see* Arousal Architecture®: Mental Headspace dimension
mental health   21, 22, 67, 78, 126, 155, 166, 169, 175, 217, 275, 284 n.7
mental well-being   78, 115, 218
mind–body connection   5, 21, 24, 36, 55, 61, 77, 85, 93, 95, 97, 177, 210, 213, 249
   for sexual satisfaction   78–81
mindfulness   4, 11–13, 16, 61, 65, 85, 88, 93, 99, 138, 167, 209–12, 214, 221, 251, 265
   based stress reduction   278 n.1 (part 1), 279 n.1 (chapter 2)
   exercises   46–50, 53
   goal of   42, 43
   Menu   53
   resources   271
   sexual   41–53
Mindfulness First Aid Kit   9, 45
mindset   11, 87, 117, 125, 128, 132, 161, 185, 217, 249, 257, 280 n.1 (chapter 4)
   beliefs, for rewriting sexual narrative   59–66
   fixed   56, 68
   growth   4, 12, 13, 16, 55–7, 67, 68, 70–2, 159
   interventions, for rewriting sexual narrative   66–72
   pleasure-based   55–74
   somatic   57, 58
   transformations, troubleshooting   70–1
   trauma-informed   57
monogamous   4, 116, 218, 226, *see also* relationship: monogamous
mirror exercise   137, 205, 258
muscle tension   18, 26, 83, 88

Nagoski, E.   208
   Come as You Are   125, 130, 282 n.14, 283 n.22
   Come Together   125, 282 n.14, 282 n.18, 283 n.20
National Asian Pacific American Women's Foundation   273
Native American peoples resources   275
National Latina Institute for Reproductive Justice   274
Native Youth Sexual Health Network   275
Neff   271
nervous system   6, 15, 18, 26, 76, 78–9, 91, 92, 97, 123, 126, 138, 146, 147, 167, 178, 211, 218
   activation and release, resilient zone for   82, 93, 94
   parasympathetic   81, 82, 84
   regulation of   24, 28, 32, 34, 36, 43, 44, 50, 53, 65, 77, 81, 83, 85, 87, 93–5, 94, 103, 105, 117, 132, 136, 137, 149, 155, 165, 166, 168, 181, 192, 193, 214, 225, 243, 251, 265
   for sexual wellness and pleasure   81–9
   sympathetic   81–5, 88–9
Nervous System Awareness and Regulation Techniques   77
neurodivergence   5, 147, 219, 271
neuropathways   4, 5, 20, 84
neuroplasticity   19, 279 n.1 (chapter 1)
neuroscience   12, 13, 23–5, 49, 173, 249
   for learning and unlearning behaviors   16–19
   for lifelong sexual transformation   15–20
neutral   27–9, 31, 33, 35, 38, 42, 43, 47, 49, 50, 52, 58, 70, 81, 94, 95, 99, 104, 105, 127, 136–8, 161, 165, 167, 168, 211, 265
   anchor   32, 37
   noticing *vs.* forcing relaxation   53
non-judgment   81, 94, 105, 135, 177

Non-Linear Sexual Response Cycle   127, 129, *129*, 130
noticing pleasant   32–4, 37–9, 58, 80, 213
numb   9, 27, 28, 31

Ogden, P.
  Trauma and the Body   23, 279 n.2
OMGYes   272
oppression   6, 25, 57, 101, 102, 114, 133, 146–9, 157, 174, 179, 233, 283 n.5
"Orange Is the New Black"   101
orgasms   18, 26, 63, 67–9, 88, 89, 102, 106, 107, 116, 118–20, 122, 124–5, 128, 129, 137, 145, 152, 153, 158, 159, 172, 195, 202, 205, 206, 212, 227, 248, 278 n.2, 282 n.9, 282 n.10, 285 n.1 (chapter 10), 286 n.1 (chapter 11)
overcoming painful sex program   183
outer labia (labia majora)   110

painful sex   9, 12, 25, 28, 75, 89–92, 137, 182–4, 209, 271
Pain Diary   258
Patient Empowerment Handout   259
parasympathetic nervous system (aka rest-and-digest system)   81, 82, 84
pelvic floor muscles   105–8, *105*
pelvic pain   137, 154, 271, 281 n.4 (chapter 6)
  chronic   280–1 n.1 (part 2), 280 n.5
  patients   207
  treatment   183
Pelvic People, The   271
penis   109–12, *111*, 116, 118, *119*, 120, 122–4, 126, 127, 133, 192, 282 n.7
penis-in-vagina (PIV) sex   56, 60, 61, 120, 133, 134, 146, 192
Perel, E.   151, 284 n.11
perfectionism   8, 64, 70–2, 89, 90, 132, 232
performance anxiety   2, 42, 58, 75
performative pleasure   160–1, 169
perineum   111

perseverance   65–6, 72, 87, 280 n.3
PFLAG   272
physical health   78, 79, 115
physiologically aroused   16, 126–8, *128*
PIV, *see* penis-in-vagina (PIV) sex
pleasant   27, 29, 31–5, 37–9, 42, 47–9, 53, 58, 61, 70, 80, 81, 88, 94, 95, 98, 99, 105, 115, 128, 137, 138, 168, 194–6, 202, 210, 211, 213, 234, 235, 241
pleasure   2, 4–6, 11, 15, 17, 23–5, 28, 30, 32–4, 41, 42, 51, 55, 63, 68, 69, 71, 75, 76, 78, 79, 81–9, 93, 96, 98, 144–6, 150, 153, 155, 157, 158, 160, 169, 174, 175, 183, 188–9, 191–6, 198, 204, 206, 210–12, 217, 218, 226, 228, 231, 233, 235, 236, 239, 241, 243–5, 252, 269, 270, 272–4, 282 n.9, 283 n.2
  anatomy of   117–25
  gems   8, 19–20, 36, 52–3, 72, 97, 135–7, 169–70
  for gender diverse folks   115–17
  motivators of   162–5
  non-sexual   32, 33
  performative   160–1
  pleasure-bombing   253
  potential   178, 179, 181, 185–7, 202, 203, 205, 209, 227, 249, 270
  science   101–39
  self-pleasure   102–5, 135
pleasure-based   2, 12, 63
  mindset   55–74
  needs   146, 179
  self-love   103
  sexual education   5–7, 12, 75, 273
polyamorous   114, 153, 218, 285 n.12
Post-Traumatic Stress Disorder (PTSD)   147, 284 n.7
Power to Decide   272
power dynamic   190, 234, 239
preface conversations   262
prejudice   5, 115, 146–8, 283 n.4
pressures of life   155–7
Principles of Pleasure, The   272

prostate   116, 122, 123
Przybylo, E.
    Asexual Erotics   235, 286 n.4
psychosomatic response   107
psychotherapy   6, 13, 22, 23, 25, 57, 71, 89, 91, 133
PTSD, *see* Post-Traumatic Stress Disorder (PTSD)

racism   5, 110, 146–9, 172
Rae   57–9
Rashatwar, S.   272
redirect to neutral or pleasant   31–3, 35, 37–9, 81, 88, 94, 136–7
regulate   24, 26, 28, 32–4, 44, 53, 65–6, 72, 77–83, 85, 88, 93–6, 99, 103, 105, 132, 136–8, 166, 193, 210, 214, 217, 223, 225
relationship   4, 17, 18, 28, 43, 46, 61, 73, 76, 80, 92, 125, 134, 143, 145–7, 158, 161, 182, 190, 191, 220, 223, 235, 262, 266–7, 283 n.6, 284 n.9
    causal   224, 227
    challenges to sexual arousal   149–53
    conflict   1, 2, 75, 149
    dissatisfaction   226
    dynamic   4, 227, 232, 239
    expectations   218
    imbalances in   150, 226, 229
    intimate   65, 225
    issues   144, 265
    maintenance   164, 165
    monogamous   1, 19, 153, 154, 218, 224, 226, 227, 285 n.12
    polyamorous   114, 285 n.12
    preferences   218, 227
    romantic   65, 284 n.10
    satisfaction   149, 151, 153, 169, 183, 218, 286 n.1 (chapter 12)
    status   148
    sexual   104, 114, 152, 224, 284 n.10
        (*see also* sexual relationship)
    styles   224, 227
    techniques   57

therapy   281 n.2 (chapter 2), 281 n.4 (chapter 4)
    uncertainties   220
    wellness   269
resistance   11–12, 29, 33, 35, 36, 45, 55, 63, 65, 66, 70, 71, 72, 82, 92–5, *94*, 97–8, 159, 175, 192, 193, 212, 217, 221, 224, 225, 279 n.5, 280 n.3, 280 n.4, 281 n.3 (chapter 5)
Resilient Zone   *82*, 93–5, *94*
responsive desire   125, 127–32, 203, 211, 264
    Arousal Architecture®   191–2
Restorative Justice Initiative
    Decolonizing Contraception   272
rewiring   4, 17, 20, 21, 24, 28, 35, 41, 43, 48, 51, 55, 72, 73, 96, 99, 168, 269
Rory   151–3

scrotum   111, 112, 120, 122
self-awareness   17, 20, 27–9, 105, 154, 155, 243
    embodied   79–81
    non-judgmental   94
self-esteem   111, 115, 227
    low   226
    sexual   9, 12
self-love   80, 102, 103, 226, 228, 252–7
self-pleasure   102–5, 135
sensations   9, 21, 22, 25–6, 43, 48, 49, 57, 59, 62, 69, 74, 80, 83, 84, 91, 93, 97, 116, 121, 124, 172, 205, 206, 232, 258
    list   27, 29, 38, 98
    neutral   32, 35, 42, 53, 58, 70, 81, 94, 95, 99, 127, 136–8, 167
    pleasant   32, 33, 35, 37–9, 42, 53, 58, 61, 70, 81, 88, 94, 95, 98, 99, 136–8, 168, 171, 178, 213, 235
    snapshot   29–32, 37–9, 70
    unpleasant   27–9, 31–3, 37, 38, 51, 136–8, 172
Sensorimotor Psychotherapy   25, 275
sensory deprivation   238

INDEX

sex drive   16, 85, 126
sex-negative   12, 18, 71, 102, 104, 117, 133, 145, 163, 174, 269
Sexological Bodyworkers   272
sex-positive   76, 145, 207, 222, 228
   counseling and education   274
SexPositive World Organization   272
Sex Surrogate Partners   272
sex therapy   6, 13, 21–5, 71, 76, 166, 228, 239
   somatic   19
sexual anatomy   5, 101–39
sexual anxiety   78, 87, 91, 207
sexual arousal   1, 2, 5, 9–10, 16, 18, 25, 26, 28, 33, 42, 62, 63, 73, 98, 102, 136, 141, 144, 155–7, 169, 170, 174, 178–9, 183, 185, 188, 191–3, 202–4, 208, 212, 217, 218, 220, 228, 231, 236, 238, 241, 251, 253, 281 n.4 (chapter 5), 282 n.15, 282 n.16, 284 n.10
   anatomy of   117–35
   anxiety and   88
   building   57, 182
   desire and   125, 126
   gender and   112–15
   healthy   32, 78, 147
   as luxury system   141
   mindfulness for increasing   51–2
   pathways   77–97
   with physiological stages   *128*
   relationship challenges to   149–53
   science of   125–35
   stress and   88–9
   system   27, 43, 117, 143, 147, 175, 177, 206, 210, 211, 225
   "technical skills" of building   57
   trauma and   89, 92
Sexual Aversion Cycle   84, 86–8, *86*, 94, 95, 142, 143, 150, 154, 162
   Arousal Architecture®   183–4, 190–1
sexual avoidance   28, 142–3, 169
sexual desire   1, 85, 126, 128, 130, 145, 232, 284 n.8, 285 n.2 (part 3)
sexual dissatisfaction   1, 11, 143, 147, 149, 191, 226
sexual dynamic   134, 227
sexual energy   155–8, 160–1, 165, 170–1, 202, 207, 219, 233, 237
sexual health wellness   272–3
Sexually Empowered Mindset Beliefs   61
sexual mindfulness   41–3, *see also* mindfulness
   arousal and   51–2
   body sandwich   48–50
   breathing and   47
   centering and   48
   grounding and   48
   movement and   48
   reasons for   44–5
   simple practices   45–8
   tips   50–1
sexual motivation   161–9
sexual narrative, mindset beliefs for rewriting   59–60
   brain functionality   62–3
   curiosity   63–4
   journey   63
   kindness   63–4
   perseverance   65–6
   sexual organ   62
sexual narrative, mindset interventions for rewriting
   growth-oriented environments   67–8
   trauma-informed   71–2
   pivoting   66–7
   shifts, imprinting   69–70
   successful sexual experiences, redefining   68–9
   transformations, troubleshooting   70–1
sexual pleasure   36, 41, 97, 104, 107, 108, 116, 134, 137, 161, 196, 198, 282 n.9, *see also* pleasure
   Arousal Architecture®   6, 178, 187, 192–3
   paradigm shift   133–6, *135*, 139, 191, 206, 241

sexual priming 152, 153
sexual relationship 104, 114, 152, 224, 284 n.10, *see also* relationship: sexual
sexual resiliency 10, 65, 78, 92, 193
　alternative possibilities, creation of 96–9
　awareness, building 97–8
　belief systems and 57–9
　building 66, 95–7, 206
　perseverance and 65–6
sexual satisfaction 3, 4, 9, 15, 16, 18, 24, 33, 44, 55, 62, 67, 68, 71, 101, 102, 104, 111, 114, 125, 133, 134, 136, 141, 144, 146, 149, 151, 153, 154, 158, 169, 170, 173–5, 177, 187, 191, 194, 201, 206, 212, 218, 220, 222, 226–8, 235, 237, 243, 252, 269, 278 n.2, 284 n.9, 284 n.10, 285 n.1 (part 3), 286 n.1 (chapter 11)
　mind–body connection for 78–81
sexual science 5, 75, 76, 125, 249
sexual self 5, 78, 173, 174, 178, 179, 181, 182, 186, 187, 204, 227, 241, 243, 245, 246, 248, 249
sexual self-awareness 17
sexual self-esteem 9, 12
sexual skills 62, 151, 241
Sexual Stimulation dimension, *see* Arousal Architecture®: Sexual Stimulation dimension
sexual transmutation 155
sexual well-being 25, 61, 104, 107, 149, 150
sexual wellness 5, 9, 12, 13, 16, 17, 23, 31, 34, 46, 57, 62, 66, 106, 125, 173, 179, 209, 212, 233, 245, 248, 252, 275
　holistic 141–72
　nervous system for 81–9, *82*
　resources, for Black and African American folks 273–4
　skills 272
Sexual Wellness Neuroscience Formula 17, 20, 27

Sexual Wellness Plans 252
sex *vs.* gender 112–15
Sexy Time Track 130, *131*, 132, 136, 151, 243
shame 2, 3, 5, 15, 16, 25, 26, 51, 56, 64, 71, 72, 75, 84, 87, 91, 96, 102, 110, 112, 117, 145, 159, 185, 190, 231, 232, 237, 248, 284 n.7
　guilt-shame spiral 20, 64, 157–8, 169
shame-based (education) 12, 101, 118
single life 154–5
sleep affirmation 58
Somatic Abolition 275
Somatic Attachment Healing 275
Somatic Experiencing 275
somatics 4, 11–13, 16, 23, 50, 51, 57–9, 61, 65, 66, 85, 88, 89, 92, 93, 96, 98, 99, 138, 161, 181, 209, 211, 213, 214, 237, 249, 251, 265, 279 n.1 (chapter 2), 279 n.3, 280 n.5
　healing practices 21, 24–34
　impact on sex 24
　resources 275
　somatic psychotherapy 22, 71
　somatic healing 22, 25
　somatic therapies 21, 22, 25, 228, 275
　timing of using 34–6
spanking 123, 238
spontaneous arousal 19, 85
spontaneous desire 125, 127, 128, 136, 191, 192, 202, 203
stigma 123, 135, 226, 231, 232, 274
stress 45, 49, 80, 81, 83, 85, 89, 93, 104, 117, 201, 217, 263, 279 n.1 (chapter 2), 280 n.5, 281 n.2 (chapter 2), 286 n.1 (chapter 12)
　chronic 82, 88
　definition of 79
　hormones 82
　management 34, 218–20
　mental 218
　reduction 2, 12, 35, 77, 78, 97, 103, 147, 278 n.1 (part 1)
　relief 165

response 79, 147, 283 n.4
successful sexual experiences, redefining 68–9
suicide prevention support 275
sympathetic nervous system (aka flight-or-fight system) 81–3, 88–9
systemic injustice 57
Symptom Tracker 258

talk therapy 22, 23
technical skills 57
testicles 112, 122
Thorpe, S. 274
threat 5, 18, 25, 26, 61, 79, 81, 82, 84, 85, 95, 107, 167
  response 89–92, 97, 166, 174, 175, 178, 190–1, 214
Tight-Lipped 271
Townes, A.
  Black Women's Pleasure Mapping 274
  #hotgirlscience 274
transgender 273, 284 n.7
trauma 18, 25, 57, 66, 115, 147, 155, 214, 279 n.2, 279 n.3, 281 n.3 (chapter 5), 283 n.5
  activation 8–9
  "Big T" 89–92
  dealing with 92
  Erotic Exploration dimension 237
  "little t" 90–1
  reprocessing 21, 23, 26, 28, 89
  response 28, 50, 78, 89, 91, 97, 166, 175
  response regulation 28
  therapist 3, 12, 23, 92, 96, 237
  therapy 71, 72, 91, 279 n.3
  treatment 23, 50, 92, 96, 209
  trigger 47, 89, 91, 92
trauma-informed 9, 26, 57, 72, 76, 237
Trauma Resource Institute 23, 91, 93, 271
Trevor Project 275
Triple Cripples 274

unlearning 16–20, 44, 80
unpleasant 18, 25, 27–9, 31–8, 48, 51, 52, 67, 80, 82, 84, 93, 94, 98, 99, 115, 136–8, 144, 154, 161, 167, 168, 172, 190, 198, 201
urethra 109–11, *109, 111*

vagina 58, 107, 109–10, *109*, 118, 121, 124
vaginal canal 109, 118, 121
vaginal opening 109, *109*, 110, 120
vaginal penetration 119
vaginismus 12, 26, 183, 214
Van der Kolk, B. A.
  Body Keeps the Score, The 23, 279 n.2
vulva 101, 109–11, *109*, 112, 118–20, 124
vulvodynia 26
  hormone-mediated 12
VWell 271

We R Native 275
World Health Organization
  stress, definition of 79

"Yes, No, Maybe" List 204, 241, 253–4, *254*, 273

ABOUT THE AUTHOR

Kayna Cassard, LMFT has been in the field of human sexuality since 2006, beginning as a Teaching Assistant for a *Sex and Intimacy Course* in her undergraduate program before continuing her studies with a Master's in Clinical Psychology. Around that same time, she became a pelvic pain patient, needing specialized help and finding insufficient support and treatment for a heartbreaking condition. Her experience with this diagnosis and the lack of adequate care marked a pivotal realization that she must integrate her education with the vital needs of pelvic pain patients. As such, Kayna dedicated her life's work to becoming a Painful Sex Specialist, Sex Therapist, and Licensed Marriage and Family Therapist.

Kayna has spent over a decade providing lectures, workshops, and presentations at universities, healthcare associations, and therapy centers. Her expertise extended to podcasts, news channels, and magazines such as *CNN*, *NPR*, *Sluts and Scholars*, *Cosmopolitan*, and *Self Magazine* as a mental health specialist and topic expert. Kayna's career continued to advance as she became a Certified Trauma Therapist, incorporating the "mind-body connection" and somatic psychotherapy into her clinical work.

Beyond her professional career, Kayna blossomed as an international acroyoga instructor and intimacy retreat leader, offering a unique perspective and enhancing her clinical skills in unconventional ways. Today, Kayna's private practice has evolved into a group practice and a modernized treatment center providing trauma-informed interventions for those dealing with sexual anxiety or pain all over the world.